AMERICAN LUNG ASSOCIATION®

Family Guide to Asthma and Allergies

✝ AMERICAN LUNG ASSOCIATION®
Family Guide to
Asthma and Allergies

The American Lung Association Asthma Advisory Group
with
Norman H. Edelman, M.D.

LITTLE, BROWN AND COMPANY
Boston   New York   London

First Edition

The American Lung Association and LifeTime Media, Inc., have exerted every effort to ensure
that the information presented in this book is accurate up to the time of publication. However, in
light of ongoing research and the constant flow of information, it is possible that new findings
may invalidate some of the data presented here. This book is meant to educate and should not be
used as an alternative to appropriate medical care. For this reason, check the safety and efficacy of
all medications and procedures with your doctor before using them.

Library of Congress Cataloging-in-Publication Data

American Lung Association family guide to asthma and allergies /
   by The American Lung Association Asthma Advisory Group, with Norman H. Edelman, M.D.
   p.   cm.
   Includes index.
   ISBN 0-316-21271-7 (hc.) ISBN 0-316-03815-6 (pbk.)
   1. Asthma — Popular works. 2. Asthma in children — Popular works.
3. Allergy — Popular works. 4. Allergy in children — Popular works.
I. Edelman, Norman H. II. American Lung Association.
RC591.A53 1997
616.2'38 — dc21   96-53497

10 9 8 7 6 5 4 3

Q-FF

PRINTED IN THE UNITED STATES OF AMERICA

Acknowledgments

The American Lung Association would like to thank the volunteers who made up the American Lung Association Asthma Advisory Group: William Busse, M.D., David Evans, Ph.D., Linda B. Ford, M.D., Robert B. Mellins, M.D., and Scott T. Weiss, M.D. Their expert help in providing information and reviewing the completed chapters was invaluable.

The American Lung Association Asthma Advisory Group

William Busse, M.D.
Professor of Medicine; Head, Allergy & Clinical Immunology
University of Wisconsin Medical School

David Evans, Ph.D.
Assistant Professor of Public Health, Department of Pediatrics
Columbia University College of Physicians and Surgeons

Linda B. Ford, M.D.
President, Board of Directors, American Lung Association
The Asthma and Allergy Center, Omaha, Nebraska

Robert B. Mellins, M.D.
Professor of Pediatrics, Columbia University College of
Physicians & Surgeons
Director, Pediatric Pulmonary Division, Babies & Children's
Hospital

Scott T. Weiss, M.D., M.S.
Professor of Medicine, Harvard Medical School
Director, Respiratory and Environmental Epidemiology,
Channing Laboratory

Contents

Introduction

Asthma is a serious lung disease that can be frightening and disabling. And for unknown reasons asthma is on the rise, affecting an estimated 14.6 million Americans. From 1982 to 1994 the number of Americans with asthma rose 84 percent. With this rise there are more people requiring hospitalization for their asthma and an increasing number of deaths from the disease.

Yet no one should suffer with asthma today. We now know how to identify what triggers asthma attacks, how to use medications to open constricted airways, and how to prevent the underlying tendency toward inflammation.

For the almost 5 million children in the United States who have asthma, controlling the disease is especially important. Research has shown that proper medical treatment and education about how to manage asthma can help children with the disease lead healthier and more active lives. Teaching these children and the adults around them how to deal with asthma also helps them perform better in school.

Allergies are one of the most common afflictions of mankind, affecting an estimated 40 million people in the United States. But allergies are nothing to sneeze at. While for some people they cause only annoying symptoms, for others they can result in serious illness, high medical costs, and even death. The good news is that you can do something about allergies—the earlier, the better. Also, the future for allergy treatment looks promising as scientists develop new medications.

New asthma treatment guidelines released in February 1997 by the federal government's National Asthma Education and Prevention Program emphasize teaching asthma self-management and prevention to patients, and stress the crucial role of the partnership between patients and physicians. The *American Lung Association Family Guide to Asthma and Allergies* can help you and your family take control of your asthma and allergies by providing the information you need to participate actively in your own health care and to work with your doctor to develop an effective plan for managing your asthma or allergies.

The *American Lung Association Family Guide to Asthma and Allergies* is one of the many ways in which the American Lung Association provides information on asthma and allergies. We also are looking ahead to the future. The American Lung Association is mounting a major initiative to find the cause or causes of asthma, which we hope will lead to a cure.

Until cures for asthma and allergies are found, the best defense against these conditions is knowing how to manage them. By following the suggestions in this book, you and your family can take charge of your asthma and allergies and lead active, healthy lives.

✝ AMERICAN LUNG ASSOCIATION®

Family Guide to Asthma and Allergies

1 / Who and Why

IF YOU OR SOMEONE IN YOUR FAMILY HAS ASTHMA OR ALLERGIES, you are not alone. An estimated 14.6 million Americans suffer from asthma, according to the American Lung Association. About one-third of those with asthma, some 4.8 million Americans, are children under age 18. And more and more people are affected by this disease: from 1982 to 1994 the rate of Americans with asthma rose 61.2 percent. While deaths are still uncommon, 5,487 people died from asthma in 1994.

The disease appears to be more common in people of all ages. Between 1982 and 1994, the rate of asthma among children aged 18 and younger climbed 72 percent; among those aged 18 to 44, asthma rates surged by 78 percent. And it is not just the young who are affected by rising asthma rates. The rate of asthma among middle-aged people, between 45 and 64, climbed nearly 40 percent, while among the elderly, aged 65 and older, rates shot up nearly 24 percent.

No one knows why the disease is affecting an increasing number of Americans, but there are some theories. Those theories come from observations about how asthma affects different groups of people. Smoking is a prime reason for asthma attacks. A recent study published by the American Lung Association found that attacks of wheezing in children could be reduced by 20 percent if parents didn't smoke in the home. One government study suggests that air pollution may be another reason for the increase in asthma; at least 63 percent of asthma sufferers live in an area where at least one federal air-quality standard is exceeded. With rates of both smoking and air pollution falling, however, researchers are faced with yet another asthma mystery that must be solved if the disease is to be brought under control.

Minority groups are hit especially hard by asthma. Nearly 61 of every 1,000 African-Americans have asthma, compared to 50 of every

1,000 white Americans. Also, African-Americans are almost four times as likely as whites to be hospitalized for asthma and three times more likely to die from the disease. Data on the prevalence of asthma in other minority groups is sketchy, with some studies indicating that the disease is slightly less common among Asians and some Hispanic groups than among whites, but slightly more common among people of Puerto Rican descent and Native Americans.

No one knows why asthma is more prevalent among African-Americans, but some clues about why they suffer more frequently from asthma may help explain why the disease is increasing in all Americans. People with asthma who live in the inner city may be exposed to more asthma triggers—such as dust mites, cockroaches, secondhand tobacco smoke, and viral infections—than are more affluent people with asthma, thus pointing to the need for all people with asthma to reduce their exposure to substances that can trigger an asthma attack. More important, deaths from asthma occur more frequently in people whose disease is poorly controlled. When people with asthma rely on visits to the hospital when their breathing has already become labored, they are far more likely to suffer severe and possibly fatal asthma attacks.

With this new understanding has come the ability to spot asthma earlier in life than ever before. Families with asthma sufferers no longer have to wait years, watching through numerous attacks, before a diagnosis is made.

This clearer understanding of the causes and effects of asthma has also spawned a new generation of medications. Gone are many of the side effects and cumbersome delivery devices that accompanied early asthma medications. In their place are pocket-sized inhalers of steroids that prevent wheezing and drugs called beta agonists that can reverse periodic breathing problems within minutes.

Attitudes about asthma also have changed. Nowadays it is the rare asthma sufferer who cannot take part in every activity that is usual for his or her age. Almost any child with asthma who wants to play even the most strenuous sport is encouraged to do so. Even hockey, football, baseball, cross-country running, and swimming are possible. People with asthma can be found among professional sports figures and Olympic athletes, some of whom will be introduced later in this book. Only rarely is a child with asthma excused from gym class. Almost all children and adults with asthma now can lead fully active lives with few restrictions.

Even as recently as 10 years ago, there was no satisfactory way to control mild to moderate asthma. But a number of recent developments have changed that situation. Asthma sufferers have tools for predicting when their disease may flare up, plus easy-to-use medications to manage the disease or to treat it after an attack. Perhaps most important, people with asthma and their families are now empowered through a better understanding of their condition.

Some of the recent developments that have made asthma a much more manageable disease are:

- *Peak Flow Meters.* These inexpensive hand-held devices can be used at home to measure the flow of air from an asthma sufferer's lungs. They can be a help in monitoring the effectiveness of a treatment and give an early warning sign that an attack is approaching.

- *Inhaled Steroids.* When used regularly, these medications can prevent asthma flare-ups in many sufferers. They are far safer than earlier oral steroid medications and can be routinely used by people who encounter breathing problems more than twice a week.

- *Inhaled Beta Agonists.* These effective drugs can relieve an acute asthma attack within minutes without causing the jitteriness and agitation that characterized earlier preparations. They come in convenient pocket-sized canisters that can be carried virtually anywhere.

- *Cromolyn and Nedocromil.* These inhaled drugs are effective in preventing bouts of wheezing in children who have chronic asthma. They have virtually no side effects.

- *Oral Steroids.* Short, 7- to 10-day courses of steroids are now judged to be a safe and effective home treatment for people who suffer from a severe episode of asthma.

- *Nonsedating Antihistamines.* These drugs can relieve much of the suffering of allergy victims without causing the daytime drowsiness that was the hallmark of earlier preparations.

- *Disease Understanding.* Asthma is a chronic condition and must be treated as such. To wait for a flare-up of wheezing before treating is to wait too long. Allergies are intimately linked to asthma. Allergic reactions in a person with asthma often precipitate an asthma attack. Discerning what a sufferer is allergic to and consciously avoiding those substances can go a long way toward preventing many asthma attacks.

- *Family Involvement.* Many families and doctors now realize that they must work with each other to achieve the best outcome for their family member with asthma. Informed families can provide the environment needed to reduce the possibility of a flare-up. Education aimed at raising family awareness of asthma and allergies, including keeping an asthma diary, is an essential part of life for families with asthma sufferers.

Alone, each of these advances is a huge step toward better control of asthma and allergies. Taken together, they are truly powerful. When a family is well informed about the condition affecting one of its members, it can make reasoned judgments about the situation. Families can control most episodes by following a plan worked out in advance with their physician.

This book will provide you with the tools needed to document the history of your asthma or allergies. It will show you how to keep a checklist of the triggers that launch your body into an attack and teach you how to monitor treatment so that you can better predict when an attack may be approaching. And it will explain how you can virtually asthma- and allergy-proof your home.

Modern medicine has made it possible for all people with asthma to control their disease and their surroundings so that they can avoid serious attacks. This book will show you how you or your family member can not only avoid becoming a statistic but live a full life with asthma.

2 / What Is Asthma?

IF SOMEONE IN YOUR FAMILY SUFFERS FROM ASTHMA, YOU PROBABLY have had the frightening experience of witnessing an asthma attack. Your child or spouse may begin to appear apprehensive and restless and may cough with each breath. Wheezing typically follows, beginning as a slight whistling sound with each exhalation and progressing to a noticeably shrill noise as your family member struggles to fill his or her lungs with air. Breathing usually becomes faster, and the sufferer appears to labor for each breath, perhaps sucking in so hard to fill the lungs that the chest appears concave. This sucking in of the chest (called retraction) occurs when a person with asthma cannot draw air into his or her lungs quickly enough. (It is most easily seen in children, who have small, flexible chests.)

While these symptoms are frightening for the observer who does not suffer from asthma, they are downright terrifying for the person with asthma who has not yet learned to control and live with the disease. People with asthma describe an attack as being choked for air. When recalling early attacks, asthma sufferers often tell of the panic they felt having to work consciously to perform something that is regularly done effortlessly: breathing.

In order to experience what breathing may be like for your family member with asthma, try this test. Begin by running in place for two minutes. Then, while pinching your nose, try breathing in enough air through a straw placed in your mouth. If you have trouble getting enough air through the narrow opening of the straw, you are simulating an asthma attack. And just as you can take the straw out of your mouth and breathe normally, better understanding of asthma and new therapies to treat the disease can allow people with asthma to breathe normally.

Asthma sufferers and their families do not have to live with regular attacks of wheezing and fright. By learning to control their disease, most people with asthma can eliminate severe attacks. And by understanding how asthma affects and changes normally operating lungs, people with asthma and their families can identify the signs of an asthma attack and know when to intervene early with medications to cut short an attack.

THE EIGHT SIGNS OF ASTHMA TROUBLE

1. *Wheezing,* beginning as a slight whistling sound and progressing to a noticeably shrill noise with each labored breath.

2. *Coughing* that gets worse over minutes to hours.

3. *Chest skin is sucked in.* In a phenomenon known as retraction, a person with asthma struggles so hard for air that the chest may appear concave and the ribs may show.

4. *Breathing out takes longer than inhaling.*

5. *Breathing is faster* as a person with asthma fights to get enough oxygen.

6. *Blue nails and lips,* especially in children.

7. *Sudden anxiety and apprehension,* especially in children.

8. *Shortness of breath.*

How Do the Lungs Work?

In order to sense what happens during an asthma attack, you must understand how the airways work under normal circumstances. The body's breathing apparatus is often referred to as the airway tree, and by the looks of it, it is aptly named. The trunk of the airway tree is the trachea, a large tube connecting the nasal passages and throat to the lungs. The trachea branches into two large roots called bronchial tubes, each feeding one of the lungs. As the bronchial tubes enter each of the lungs, they branch off into smaller airways, or bronchioles, the complex root system of the airway tree. At the end of each bronchiole is a pouch of airway sacs, called alveoli, each resembling a small floret of cauliflower. It is within the alveoli that the true work of breathing takes place.

The lungs are a wonderfully engineered, intricately designed mechanism for getting oxygen to the blood. When we breathe, air flows down the trachea into the bronchial tubes and bronchioles and collects in the 300 million alveoli we have in our lungs. Tiny blood vessels flowing by the alveoli pick up oxygen and carry it throughout the body, nourishing all our tissues. The air left in the alveoli, which now contains "waste" gases, leaves the body when we exhale.

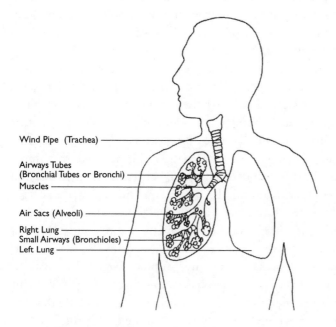

Wind Pipe (Trachea)

Airways Tubes
(Bronchial Tubes or Bronchi)
Muscles

Air Sacs (Alveoli)

Right Lung
Small Airways (Bronchioles)
Left Lung

The airway tree allows air to flow into the lungs, where oxygen is captured.

What Can Go Wrong?

When all is working according to plan, the system operates flawlessly. Air flows effortlessly down relaxed, wide-open airways, filling millions of air sacs with oxygen, which is whisked away by the blood system. Unfortunately, many things can go wrong with this system. Asthma, emphysema, chronic obstructive pulmonary disease, lung cancer, cystic fibrosis, severe bouts with influenza, and other respiratory infections can all affect how efficiently the lungs get oxygen to the bloodstream.

What goes wrong in a person with asthma has everything to do with how asthma redesigns the lungs. Some scientists believe that people with asthma actually have a smaller root system to their bronchial tree; that is, the disease may cause the lungs to develop more slowly, leaving fewer and smaller bronchioles and alveoli to fill with life-sustaining air. It is not known whether this occurs at birth, because a person with asthma has inherited some asthma gene, or whether early asthma attacks or infections during childhood choke the lungs and prohibit them from growing normally. What is known is that a smaller airway-tree root system alone is not enough to cause asthma.

Asthma is a disease that causes the airways in the lungs to be "twitchy." This twitchiness causes the airways to become temporarily constricted or even blocked when a person with asthma comes into contact with an asthma trigger. An asthma trigger can be anything from cigarette smoke or cold air to exercise or allergens. (More information about asthma triggers is given in chapter 3.) This tendency for the airways to overreact is often present from infancy. In fact, most researchers agree that the tendency to develop asthma is genetic, that is, passed on from one generation to the next. Geneticists are actively trying to locate which gene or combination of genes leads to asthma, but as yet, this link has eluded detection. What is known is that the majority of people with asthma also have a condition known as allergic rhinitis, or hay fever, meaning they are allergic to pollen, grasses, molds, and other airborne allergens. These allergens can trigger an asthma attack, or they can leave the lungs inflamed and thus so close to an asthma attack that exposure to any asthma trigger can lead to wheezing and breathlessness. The observation that many people with asthma also have allergic rhinitis has led scientists to conclude that the gene or genes responsible for asthma are located near the gene or genes that cause allergic disease. Thus, if you inherit the mechanism responsible for allergies, you are likely to inherit the genes that cause both.

The road to finding a genetic or hereditary link to asthma, however, is a long one. Asthma is not a simple disease, and recent research indicates that a number of genes may be needed to cause the condition. It could be that in order to inherit asthma you must receive asthma genes from both parents. That may explain why some families in which one spouse has asthma have children who are not affected by the disease. Or it could mean that only one parent need donate asthma genes in order to produce a child with the disease but that a number of specific genes must all be donated at the same time.

Airway twitchiness in asthma means that the bronchioles and alveoli can become narrowed or blocked. This can happen in three ways during an asthma attack. First, the muscles encircling the airways tighten, narrowing the air passageway within. Second, the reaction causes fluid, blood cells, and irritating chemicals to enter the bronchioles. This in turn causes the lining of the airways to become inflamed, thus narrowing the air passage. Finally, in response to this inflammation, mucous glands in the bronchioles secrete more mucus than usual, causing the airways to become plugged or blocked.

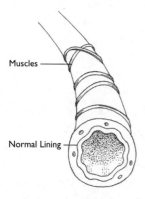

In people without asthma, the bronchi remain relaxed and wide open, allowing air to enter the lungs.

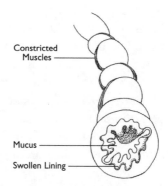

Asthma attacks occur when muscles surrounding the bronchi tighten, and when the tubes fill with sticky mucus.

Much has been learned about asthma in recent years, but nothing is more important than the observation that asthma is a disease of airway inflammation. By this physicians mean that people with asthma have chronically inflamed airways that are ever prone to become twitchy and constricted after exposure to an asthma trigger. It is as if the airways of people with asthma are lying in wait for trouble. They stay poised at the edge of a cliff, where the slightest exposure to an asthma trigger can push them over the edge and cause them to launch into a full-fledged asthma attack.

This means that asthma is both a chronic and an episodic disease. The chronic part means that the lungs in people with asthma are always inflamed. The inflammation is the result of a constant release by the body of irritating cells and chemicals called cytokines that confuse the lungs and cause them to become swollen, much as if they were responding to some infection by rejecting it. Cytokines cause cells within the lungs to break down and release a host of other chemicals that lead to the inflammation. The episodic part of asthma means that the chronically inflamed lungs can be kicked over the edge and will constrict beyond the point where normal breathing is possible. Episodic asthma, or an asthma attack, usually occurs after exposure to an asthma trigger, causing the classic wheezing and coughing usually associated with asthma.

In other words, asthma can be characterized as a disease with two phases. The early phase begins when the lungs are left chronically swollen and inflamed because of repeated exposure to an irritant. Inflammation-causing irritants are known as asthma promoters. Common asthma promoters are cigarette smoke, air pollution, respiratory infections, influenza, allergens, or other substances that irritate the lungs of people with asthma and cause them to be chronically inflamed. The underlying inflammation may not be enough to cause breathing problems, but it is enough to leave asthma sufferers on the verge of wheezing. Once a person with inflamed airways encounters an asthma trigger, he or she launches into an attack of wheezing.

The realization that asthma is a disease of airway inflammation has led to a complete revision in how the disease is diagnosed and treated. New asthma medications are now being designed to reduce the early phase of asthma, the chronic lung inflammation, so that attacks of wheezing can be prevented. (Information about medications to treat asthma is provided in chapters 4 and 5.)

Diagnosing Asthma

Even the slightest symptoms associated with asthma should be taken seriously. Many doctors believe that a significant number of people with asthma never get proper treatment because they do not recognize the signs of asthma and consequently do not seek medical attention. If you or someone in your family coughs regularly or experiences tightness in the chest, shortness of breath, or wheezing, you should see a doctor. Even if these symptoms occur only occasionally, they should not be ignored. For instance, you or a family member may cough only when playing or exercising; wheezing may be present only when you are gardening, doing yard work, or trying to sleep at night; and shortness of breath may occur only around a smoker or at work. Yet all these symptoms may indicate asthma.

Asthma can be a difficult disease to diagnose because it can resemble other diseases such as emphysema, bronchitis, heart disease, and some respiratory infections. For that reason, it may be underdiagnosed, with some people who have asthma going undetected and therefore undertreated for years. If you think that you or someone in your family has asthma, tell your doctor. The first thing he or she will do is get a detailed medical history. You can assist your doctor by tracking the history of the asthma attacks.

Your doctor will start by asking about what kinds of symptoms you are experiencing: do you cough frequently and do you wheeze or often experience shortness of breath. You will be asked about feelings of chest tightness and how much saliva you produce. The doctor will also want to know about conditions known to be associated with asthma, such as a constantly runny or stuffy nose or chronic skin rashes.

When these symptoms appear is also important in diagnosing asthma. Because many people with asthma also have hay fever, they often experience more difficulty breathing during certain times of the year, when increases in pollen act as the kick that already inflamed airways need to launch into an attack of wheezing. If you have difficulty breathing every spring or fall or when you cut the grass, for instance, chances are you are having asthma attacks caused by breathing irritating amounts of pollen or grasses. Your doctor also will want to know if you have trouble breathing at night. That's because, in many people, asthma attacks seem to worsen during sleep.

The ability of your lungs to function diminishes during sleep (whether or not you have nightly asthma). Lung function typically is lowest about 4:00 A.M. For asthma sufferers, this drop in lung function at night is more pronounced. One study by asthma researchers in Denver found that the lung function in people with asthma is about 8 percent poorer at 4:00 A.M. than the lung function in people who do not have asthma. The same study found that among asthma sufferers, those who experience frequent bouts of nighttime wheezing have airways that are eight times more likely to become constricted than do those who are not bothered by nighttime symptoms. This could mean that people with asthma who have frequent attacks of nighttime wheezing are more likely to be bothered by asthma triggers when they are asleep.

Once your doctor has taken a complete history of the symptoms affecting you, he or she may then follow a plan for diagnosing and treating asthma developed by doctors working on the federal government's National Asthma Education and Prevention Program. In that plan, which was designed to take some of the guesswork out of diagnosing asthma, your doctor begins by administering tests to determine the degree of your airway obstruction. These tests are performed in a doctor's office on a machine called a spirometer. The spirometer measures how efficiently the lungs are working by gauging how quickly and with how much force a person with asthma can exhale one full breath of air. These measurements are the only accurate way to determine the level of lung function in a person with asthma. Your doctor will ask you to blow as hard as you can into a tube connected to the spirometer. The force of that breath will be calculated and give the doctor a good idea of how obstructed the lungs are.

If results from this test indicate that you have some degree of airway obstruction, your physician will administer an inhaled drug called a beta agonist, or bronchodilator. These types of drugs can quickly reverse airway obstruction and are used when people with asthma have an asthma attack. After the drug takes effect, your doctor will once again administer the spirometry test. If the results on the second test are better than on the first test after use of the inhaled anti-asthma drug, a diagnosis of asthma is made.

Not everyone with asthma has airway obstruction at the time he or she visits the doctor. It's much like that painful tooth that never seems to hurt once you get to the dentist. If spirometry tests show no signs of airway obstruction, your doctor will probably ask you to measure your own airway function at home over the following two to four weeks using a hand-held gauge called a peak flow meter. Recommended for all people with greater than mild asthma, the peak flow meter is an easy and accurate way to measure how efficiently the lungs in a person with asthma are operating and, when used regularly, may help predict when an asthma attack is approaching. (More details on using a peak flow meter and keeping a diary of airway obstruction are presented in chapter 4.) If after you monitor your airways at home your doctor finds indications of airway obstruction, he or she will administer the inhaled beta agonist drug and retest you on the spirometer. Once again, if after using the inhaled drug the test results improve, your doctor will determine that you have asthma. However, if the results of your home use of a peak flow meter indicate that you do not have airway obstruction, your doctor will start looking for other diseases that may be causing your wheezing and coughing. These diseases include emphysema, heart disease, bronchitis, and some respiratory infections.

Some people have asthma that is so erratic or intermittent that the results of both spirometry tests and peak flow monitoring do not give their doctor enough clues to make a proper diagnosis. In these cases, the doctor may ask the patient to undergo another test called a bronchoprovocation test. In this test, the doctor administers drugs that cause the airways of people with asthma to go into a mild spasm. It's as if these drugs trick the airways into thinking they have been exposed to some asthma trigger. If the patient starts coughing or wheezing after receiving these drugs and the lung function changes, the doctor can accurately diagnose asthma. Since bronchoprovocation tests can cause

TRACKING YOUR ASTHMA HISTORY

What Kinds of Symptoms *(Check all that apply.)*
- ❑ Coughing
- ❑ Wheezing
- ❑ Shortness of breath
- ❑ Chest tightness

When Symptoms Occur *(Check all that apply.)*
- ❑ Year-round
- ❑ Seasonal (Note season.)
- ❑ At night
- ❑ During particular outdoor activities, such as mowing the lawn, raking leaves, gardening, or exercising

Factors Leading to Symptoms *(Check all that apply.)*
- ❑ Irritants, especially tobacco smoke
- ❑ Respiratory infection
- ❑ Cold air
- ❑ Environmental allergens such as pollen, mold, house dust, animal dander
- ❑ Chemicals at the workplace
- ❑ Exercise

When Asthma Symptoms Began *(Fill in each blank.)*

Age when symptoms started: _____

Progress of disease since: _____

Previous diagnoses or medications: _____

Home Environment *(Check all that apply, and fill in the blanks.)*
- ❑ Smoker in home
- ❑ Animals in home

Home age: _____

Type of heating, including periodic use of wood-burning stove:
_____

Description of patient's bedroom, including type of pillow, bedding, and floor covering: _____

Family History

Other family members or relatives with asthma or allergies:
_____
_____
_____

asthma attacks, they should be performed only in a doctor's office or in the hospital. If your doctor asks you to take the test, there is no reason for worry. He or she will have on hand medications that can quickly reverse the asthma attack and restore normal breathing.

To determine how severe your asthma is, your doctor will want to know how many times a week you launch into an attack of wheezing. Determining the severity of asthma is important because it helps the doctor gauge what types of asthma medications can best control your attacks. To better tailor the right amount and type of medication needed to control and prevent asthma attacks, specialists in respiratory medicine have classified asthma into varying degrees of severity; doctors classify how severe a person's asthma is by determining how often he or she has attacks of wheezing and by checking the measurements taken on a peak flow meter.

Once your doctor has taken a medical history, learned how often your asthma attacks occur, and measured airway obstruction on a peak flow meter, he or she will determine the severity of your asthma. The mildest form of asthma is known as intermittent or mild asthma. People with this form of asthma may experience wheezing and coughing lasting less than one hour and occurring no more than twice a week. They typically have no asthma symptoms between attacks and may have flare-ups at night up to twice a month. Their lungs operate at 80 percent of what is considered normal when measured on a peak flow meter or on more sophisticated equipment in a doctor's office.

Moderate asthma occurs in people whose asthma symptoms happen more than twice a week and may last for several days. Wheezing and coughing may be severe enough to interfere with normal activities and even disturb sleep. People with this category of asthma have lungs that perform at between 60 and 80 percent of normal.

People with severe asthma have continuous asthma symptoms that limit their activity and frequently disturb their sleep. They also may require occasional hospitalization to control their breathing. People with this form of asthma have lungs that operate at less than 60 percent of normal.

If you and your doctor perform an adequate workup, you will learn whether or not you have asthma. Far from being bad news, a diagnosis of asthma is the first step toward controlling the disease, preventing attacks, and leading a perfectly normal life. Once you know how severe a case of asthma is affecting you, your doctor will prescribe drugs that prevent most attacks and cut short the few flare-ups that still happen. You will understand what factors cause an asthma attack, and armed with that knowledge, you will be able to avoid or minimize your exposure to these triggers. With the help of your doctor, you also will be able to develop an asthma emergency plan to follow should you get into real trouble breathing. Asthma emergency plans are key to controlling asthma because they can guide you through the steps you must take during an asthma attack. (Some sample asthma emergency plans are provided in chapters 4 and 5.)

Asthma Myths

Now that you know what asthma is, let's look at what it is not. Here are some of the many common myths about asthma and reasons you should not believe them.

Asthma is all in your head. Because asthma sufferers may have an attack when they are under stress or emotional turmoil, some people have held that the disease itself is psychosomatic. It is not. Asthma is real. It starts in the airways, not in the head. New understandings about the interplay between the mind and body have led to explanations about why psychological stress can cause underlying diseases to worsen. Stress causes many chemical changes in the body; some of these changes include the excessive release of chemicals and cells that can irritate or constrict the linings of the bronchial tree, thus mimicking the beginnings of an asthma attack. Stress can therefore act as an asthma trigger, causing already existing asthma to worsen. That is a far cry from saying the disease itself is all in your head.

You will grow out of asthma. If you are diagnosed with asthma, it is likely you will have it for life. Asthma is almost always a chronic disease. As people with asthma grow older and become more accustomed to their disease, they are often able to anticipate an impending asthma attack and take steps to prevent it or lessen its severity. In a sense, the longer you have asthma, the better you become at controlling and living with it. In addition, the growth spurt during adolescence may increase the size of the airways and decrease the chance that they will become obstructed. Therefore, asthma in adults often causes fewer problems than in children. But the underlying disease is always there and must always be treated if a person with asthma is to live a full and healthy life.

In one study published by the American Lung Association, Dutch and American researchers found that of 350 children first treated for asthma when they were between the ages of 8 and 12, 85 percent of females and 78 percent of males continued to have symptoms 15 years later. As adults, many people in the study had asthma symptoms that were less severe than when they were children, but doctors think that the probable reason is that they became more familiar with their disease and how to control it. As children grow, their airways become larger and their breathing problems may become less frequent, but the underlying tendency for the airways and lungs to become inflamed is a pattern that persists throughout life.

Nobody dies from asthma anymore. Asthma is a serious disease that unfortunately causes about 5,000 deaths a year in the United States alone. And deaths from asthma are on the rise. Nobody knows why more people are dying from asthma, but some studies indicate that the people with asthma who are most likely to die from the disease do not get adequate preventive treatment. If you suspect that you or someone in your family has asthma, you should see a doctor, who can diagnose the disease and prescribe medications to control breathing. There is no reason for anyone with asthma to die from the disease, and with proper care that may someday be the case.

Asthma is a periodic disease that causes only occasional wheezing. Asthma is a chronic disease that is present even when people with asthma are breathing normally. The disease alters the airways of sufferers, leaving them inflamed and prone to choke off the air supply. Only with this understanding can people with asthma take the appropriate measures to reduce asthma attacks and lessen their severity when they occur. To think of asthma as being present only when a person with the disease is wheezing would be the same as thinking that high cholesterol levels do not matter until a person has a heart attack.

Most people with asthma do not need medications. Virtually every person with asthma, no matter how mild the disease may be, can benefit from asthma medications. Proper and regular use of asthma medications is the only way to control the disease. And with regular medication use, most people with asthma can lead lives no different from those of people without this disease. Much progress has been made in the field of asthma drugs over the last few years: new inhaled steroids can prevent most asthma attacks from ever occurring; inhaled beta agonists can quickly reverse attacks; and antihistamines can prevent most allergic reactions to asthma triggers.

If you want to breathe easier, move to the desert. Most people with asthma also have allergies to pollen and molds, and many react to cold air. The "hot, dry air" theory grew out of the observation that these offending allergens are far less common in the heat of the American Southwest. While some people with asthma appear to benefit from climate changes, there are many things you can do to avoid or control these asthma triggers without relocating the entire family. Antihistamines can reduce allergic reactions to pollen, grasses, and molds. Wearing a scarf over your mouth in the cold can heat and moisturize air before it is breathed in. Asthma is a disease that can be lived with anywhere, so unless you like the climate and cacti, moving to the desert is not likely to help.

3 / The Triggers and Promoters of Asthma and Allergies

PEOPLE WITH ASTHMA HAVE AIRWAYS THAT ARE PREDISPOSED to becoming inflamed, constricted, and blocked; these features are what cause the classic asthma signs of wheezing, coughing, and breathlessness. If you or someone in your family has asthma, however, you know that most people with the disease do not have trouble breathing all the time. They breathe normally most of the time and are unhampered by asthma attacks during most days and nights.

But when asthma strikes, it may seem as though it has crept up for no apparent reason. One minute you, your spouse, or your child may be reading, sleeping, playing, or exercising without a thought given to breathing; the next minute a telltale wheeze may appear, progressing to shortness of breath and, soon after, a full-fledged asthma attack. Asthma attacks do not, however, start without reason. And once you understand what can trigger an attack—and what can predispose the airways to constrict when exposed to asthma triggers—you will be on the road to controlling your disease.

Asthma is a disease of promoters and triggers. Without these, no person with asthma ever would experience bouts of breathing problems. Promoters cause the hypersensitive lungs of people with asthma to become inflamed. Asthma triggers come into play by causing an asthma attack in people with already inflamed airways. People with asthma can help control their disease by limiting their exposure to these promoters and triggers—that is, by controlling their environment.

One of the first cases of using environmental controls to reduce asthma attacks can be dated to 1552, when the longtime asthma sufferer Archbishop Hamilton of Saint Andrews in Scotland summoned the physician Girolamo Cardano to help ease his wheezing. In addition to prescribing a proper diet and exercise regimen, Cardano removed a leather pillow and feather bed from the archbishop's bedroom. The patient's breathing improved dramatically. Cardano probably succeeded because he reduced the archbishop's exposure to asthma triggers, namely, the pillow and the feather bed. Feathers and dander from such animals as cats and dogs are well-known asthma triggers. The archbishop's leather pillow may also have acted as an asthma trigger by collecting dust. Tiny insects that live in dust, called house dust mites, are another common asthma trigger.

How Triggers and Promoters Work

The airways of people with asthma are abnormal. They are more likely to react to inhaled substances by causing the constriction of the muscles surrounding the bronchioles, thus narrowing the air passageway within. The airways of people with asthma are also supercharged with cells and chemicals that initiate the early phase of asthma, known as chronic inflammation. When these cells and chemicals are activated by asthma promoters and triggers, they cause irritating fluids to enter the bronchioles, irritating and inflaming them and thus blocking the passageway further. In response to this inflammation, mucous glands in the airways secrete more mucus than usual, causing the airways to become plugged or blocked. Alone, each one of the mechanisms can cause an asthma attack. Together, they may lead to prolonged or severe bouts of breathing problems.

As discussed in chapter 2, most people with asthma also have allergies, most commonly allergic rhinitis (or hay fever). Doctors do not know exactly what percentage of people with asthma also have allergies, but they are becoming more convinced that these two conditions occur together very frequently. However, people with asthma do not have to have allergen contact for their airways to become constricted and inflamed. Some asthma triggers are not allergens, yet they can still irritate the airways. These substances can directly irritate the airway tree and cause the body to respond to this irritation by secreting excess amounts of mucus and constricting the bronchioles. Air pollution, stress, emotions, cold air, exercise, odors, and certain respiratory infections are asthma promoters and triggers that do not cause an allergic reaction but can still lead to asthma attacks. Tobacco smoke can act as an airway irritant in people with asthma and also can stimulate the allergic response in people with both asthma and allergies. (The link between asthma and allergies is discussed further in chapter 7.)

"Billy"

Billy's story really begins before birth. His parents, Barbara and Matt, have asthma and allergies, and they knew there was a strong chance that they would have a child with these conditions. While Barbara and Matt both have allergic rhinitis, or hay fever, Barbara's asthma is the more severe.

Because they were educated about asthma and allergies, Barbara and Matt did everything they could to prevent the disease from taking hold in their child. Neither parent smoked; Billy's room was never cluttered with stuffed animals or other furry toys; there were no animals in the home; his bedroom had no carpeting and was furnished with mostly hardwood furniture that could be kept clean and dusted.

Billy's first sign of breathing problems came when he was about six months old. He was lying on the floor playing when Barbara heard that familiar, telltale wheeze. "I knew right away what it was because we were prepared for this," Barbara says. "I knew he was not in grave danger, but I also knew he had to see a doctor and get treated. In this respect we were lucky because we already knew about asthma. I can only imagine how terrifying it must be for parents who know nothing about this to suddenly be confronted with a child who is wheezing."

The first episode was mild and treatable with some liquid beta-adrenergic drugs to open Billy's clogged airways. But Barbara and Matt found that the biggest problem was convincing the doctor that Billy's problems might be due to asthma. "He just couldn't believe that Billy would have symptoms at such a young age or that we could spot the problem ourselves," Barbara says. By the time Billy was about two years old, he was on maintenance doses of liquid theophylline and was prone to more and more allergies. He had trouble in the spring and fall when pollen and mold spores filled the air, and he was beginning to have bouts of nighttime asthma.

Barbara and Matt struggled to keep the house as dust free as possible and to try to reduce Billy's exposure to other asthma triggers. But Billy had never had a set of skin tests to determine which allergens could trigger an asthma attack. "So we were basically operating on guesswork, doing our best to reduce his exposure to what we thought were causing attacks," Barbara says.

The defining moment came when Billy was about four years old and needed his first course of oral steroids to reverse a rather severe asthma attack. "I remember that it was the first time I was really terrified about his asthma," Barbara says. The attack started like many others. Billy began wheezing while playing. Barbara gave him some liquid beta-adrenergic drug to open his clogged airways, but Billy kept wheezing. At the hospital the doctors gave Billy an injection of epinephrine, which restored his breathing for a while, but even that didn't last. "So they started him on a course of prednisone, and I knew then and there that his disease was getting worse and we were going to have to take some dramatic action," Barbara says.

That action came in the form of a visit to a specialist in asthma and allergies. The specialist told Barbara and Matt that despite their best efforts to reduce Billy's exposure to asthma triggers, he still had probably inherited the genes responsible for asthma and allergies. The doctor gave Billy a set of skin tests that determined he was allergic to a number of seasonal pollens and mold spores. Billy began a series of allergy immunotherapy injections to desensitize his body to the allergens and perhaps reduce the chance that they would cause asthma attacks. And his theophylline maintenance dose was increased. The doctor also told Billy's parents to buy a nebulizer and face mask so that Billy could get inhaled drugs to open his airways during an attack.

Although the nebulizer, theophylline, and immunotherapy injections helped, Billy still had breakthrough asthma attacks, sometimes quite severe. Barbara would crush his prednisone pills and mix them in a little applesauce to make them easier to take. "The biggest temptation during this time was to treat Billy like he was different," says Barbara. "We were so worried about him that we wanted to give in to everything he wanted. But Matt and I decided that we didn't want to make Billy think he was different from other kids his age, so we treated him just like we would have if he didn't have asthma."

With the advent a few years later of pocket-sized inhalers of steroids and beta-adrenergic drugs, Billy's asthma became much better. At seven he is able to control his own disease by taking an inhaled steroid three times a day and using his beta-adrenergic drug only when he is wheezing. Now when he is playing and has trouble breathing, he just takes a few minutes and uses his inhaler and is soon back in action with the other kids. "It's really amazing to see, but Billy is growing up just like any other child. There is nothing he can't do, and he really takes his asthma in stride," says Barbara. "It was just a matter of getting the right medication schedule and developing a plan that he could stick to." ❑

Allergic Asthma

In order to understand how allergies can promote and trigger an asthma attack, let's look at our immune system, which responds to infections and diseases by initiating a defense mechanism that blocks and then works to kill invading viruses or bacteria.

In some people with asthma, a unique antibody, IgE, is overproduced in response to allergens. It is hypersensitive, responding to substances in the body that do not pose a threat, or overresponding to relatively innocuous substances with a full-scale attack when a smaller assault may be all that is needed. It may be that people with asthma are simply born with IgE systems that are predisposed to overproduce this allergic antibody. If this is the case, some doctors believe that exposure to allergens such as tobacco smoke, dust mites, animal dander, and other asthma triggers very early in life may permanently shift the IgE system in people with asthma into overdrive.

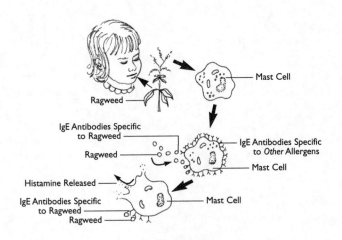

*When people with asthma are exposed to an allergen,
mast cells release chemicals that cause asthma and allergy attacks.*

A hypersensitive IgE system responds to allergens inhaled into the lungs. People with allergies have a specific type of IgE antibody for each substance to which they are allergic. The IgE antibodies are attached to another part of the immune system called the mast cells. If you or your family member is allergic to certain tree pollens, there are IgE antibodies for those tree pollens lying in wait on the mast cells. When these IgE antibodies attract and latch on to allergic substances, they trigger the mast cells to release a host of chemicals called cytokines, or inflammatory mediators.

Chief among these cytokines and inflammatory mediators are the chemicals histamine and leukotriene. These substances irritate the sensitive lining of the airway tree, just as repeatedly scratching an insect bite irritates your skin. The airway tree responds to this irritation by becoming inflamed and overproducing mucus. This inflammation and mucus may not be enough to cause a person with asthma to wheeze and cough, but it is enough to leave his or her airways chronically inflamed. The key to controlling asthma rests in reducing this airway-tree inflammation before it causes an attack of wheezing. (More information about anti-inflammation asthma medications is given in chapters 4 and 5.)

ASTHMA PROMOTERS AND TRIGGERS

Promoters

Allergies
    Hay fever, or allergic rhinitis
    Molds
    Grass pollens
    Tree pollens
    Weed pollens
    House dust and house dust mites
    Cockroaches
    Pets, most commonly dogs, cats, and birds
    Certain food additives

Tobacco smoke

Colds and respiratory infections

Triggers

Tobacco smoke

Exercise

Weather
    Wind
    Cold air
    Dramatic changes in weather

Medications
    Aspirin
    Certain drugs used to treat high blood pressure
        and some heart conditions

Emotions
    Stress
    Crying
    Laughing
    Yelling
    Hyperventilating

Irritants
    Aerosol sprays
    Odors, perfumes
    Smoke from wood-burning stoves and cooking

Asthma Promoters

Asthma promoters can include tobacco smoke, respiratory infections, some substances encountered on the job, and allergens, any of which can cause the lungs of people with asthma to become inflamed. Many of these substances may also perform double duty, working as asthma triggers and causing attacks of wheezing in people with already inflamed lungs. The following are some of the more common asthma promoters.

Tobacco smoke is one of the most dangerous asthma promoters. Of course, people with asthma should not smoke cigarettes, but secondhand smoke is also dangerous to them. Numerous studies have found that when one family member smokes in the home, other family members with asthma have longer and more frequent asthma attacks. Cigarette smoke is an irritant that acts as both an asthma promoter (causing chronic airway inflammation) and an asthma trigger (tripping inflamed airways over the edge by leading to constriction of the bronchioles and wheezing).

Respiratory infections are the most common promoters of chronic lung inflammation and asthma attacks in children. Influenza viruses, cold bugs, and the respiratory syncytial virus (a common childhood infection known as RSV) invade the nose, throat, lungs, and other parts of the airway tree. Viruses can cause airway inflammation and asthma attacks in a number of ways. They can work by increasing the amount of inflammatory chemicals released by mast cells. As we have learned, these chemicals cause the lungs to become inflamed and secrete excess amounts of mucus. Because respiratory viruses can last for many days, they also can act as asthma triggers by repeatedly acting on mast cells after the airways already become inflamed.

Some doctors believe that viruses also may alter the way the lungs respond to asthma stimuli for some time after the infection itself has cleared. Viruses may reduce the number and sensitivity of areas in the bronchioles that are the targets of beta-agonist asthma medications. That means that a person with asthma who has a respiratory infection may be less likely to be helped by some inhaled asthma medications.

It should be noted that antibiotic medications such as penicillin and erythromycin do not kill viruses. These medications therefore do not help in treating asthma attacks promoted and triggered by viruses.

Allergies to substances like pollen and molds can be potent triggers of asthma attacks. Many people with asthma also have an allergy known as allergic rhinitis, or more commonly, as hay fever. People with allergic rhinitis have IgE systems that treat these inhaled allergens like invading forces. Their bodies recognize the pollen, which then stimulates their mast cells to release the inflammatory chemicals, triggering an asthma attack. The main chemical released by mast cells in people with allergic rhinitis is histamine, which, in addition to triggering an asthma attack, also causes runny noses and watery eyes.

House dust is the home for tiny insects called house dust mites, which also can trigger an asthma attack. The feces of these insects are a known allergen, and many people with asthma are allergic to them. The feces of these insects, which themselves are so small they can be seen only under a microscope, are inhaled into the lungs when a person breathes in tiny dust particles. Once in the lungs of a person with asthma, the feces are recognized and attacked by the body's IgE antibodies. The National Cooperative Inner City Asthma Study, a survey of more than 1,500 children with asthma in New York, Cleveland, Baltimore, Washington, Chicago, St. Louis, and Detroit, found that 23 percent of inner-city children with asthma reacted to dust mites.

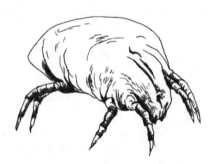

*The feces of **dust mites**, tiny insects that live in dust particles, are among the most potent allergens known.*

Cockroaches, in addition to being the bane of many urban dwellers, are a potent asthma trigger. Any person who has ever lived in a city apartment knows that for every roach you see, there are hundreds of others hiding behind walls and in cracks and crevices. Because these little creatures often live and die out of sight, people rarely have the ability to clean up their decomposing bodies. In time, dead cockroaches turn into dust, which is aerosolized in fine particles just like house dust. These tiny roach particles are inhaled into the lungs, where they excite the IgE antibodies and trigger an asthma attack. About 36 percent of inner-city children with asthma are sensitive to cockroaches, according to the National Cooperative Inner City Asthma Study.

Pets, while lovable and cuddly, can trigger an asthma attack. The dander of dogs and cats is an especially potent inhaled allergen that can trigger already inflamed lungs into launching an attack of wheezing. Rodents, such as hamsters, can also be a problem. The dander also acts as an asthma promoter by causing chronic airway inflammation.

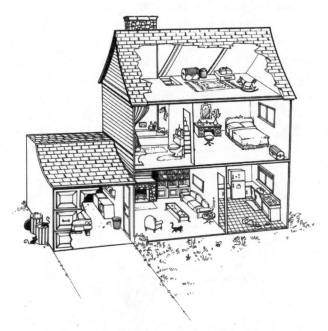

The home can be full of asthma triggers, including indoor pets, dust, molds, cooking odors, and scented soaps.

Asthma Triggers

Once chronically inflamed, the airways of people with asthma are primed for an asthma attack. It is then that asthma triggers can do the most harm by signaling the airways to constrict beyond the point where normal breathing is possible. If not for the underlying inflammation, the effect of asthma triggers would not be as great. Think of two balloons, one with no air in it and the other inflated to the point just before it is ready to pop. Now take a pin and gently prick both balloons. Certainly the pin can put a hole in the deflated balloon, but you have to press a little. But just touch the pin to the already overinflated balloon and, bang! That's how asthma triggers operate. In a person with chronic lung inflammation, just a little exposure to an asthma trigger can cause an attack.

Asthma triggers can be cold air, exercise, air pollution, odors, weather changes, emotions, and smoke. Even the simple acts of laughing, yelling, or crying can be asthma triggers. The following are some common asthma triggers and how they may work to cause an attack. (For tips on how to trigger-proof your life, see chapter 6.)

Exercise is one of the most common triggers of asthma. About 80 percent of people with asthma complain of chest tightness, coughing, or wheezing when they exercise. This does not mean that people with asthma should not exercise. What it does mean is that their underlying airway inflammation must be adequately controlled. Exercise triggers asthma attacks because it requires the participant to breathe fast and hard. This causes the temperature in the bronchioles to be lowered as air passes through them at a greater rate, and tends to make the airways drier. Some people with asthma may have exercise-induced symptoms even if their lungs are not chronically inflamed. This type of exercise-induced asthma usually appears within about five minutes of beginning exercise and subsides when the activity is stopped. A common form of exercise-induced asthma appears within the five minutes immediately after stopping exercise.

People with properly controlled asthma can participate in any sport or exercise they wish. Professional athletes with asthma are found in numerous sports, from baseball to track and field to swimming. Many doctors believe that regular exercise combined with controlled asthma may actually result in better long-term breathing. And the benefits from exercise far outweigh any risks when a person with asthma is receiving proper preventive medications.

Cooking odors have long been suspected as an asthma trigger. Certain types of cooking (such as heavy frying or broiling) may produce excess amounts of kitchen smoke, and this smoke can act as an airway irritant.

Indoor air pollution can exist in many forms. Smoke from wood-burning stoves, fumes from gas and oil furnaces, perfumes, aerosol sprays, and cooking odors can all irritate the airways of people with asthma. When these are combined with such allergens as dust mites, cockroaches, and pet dander, the home environment becomes a significant source of asthma triggers. One recent observation holds that many of the features of the modern home that are synonymous with creature comforts may be increasing the number of asthma triggers within the walls you call home.

Some doctors say that wall-to-wall carpeting, better insulation, double-pane windows, and sealed energy-efficient houses may be turning homes into breeding grounds for asthma triggers. Part of what makes the modern energy-efficient home save energy is that less outside air flows through leaky windows and poorly insulated walls. While less drafty home construction is good for energy conservation, it may be bad for people with asthma, since indoor asthma triggers no longer have the chance to be ventilated to the outside air. Add wall-to-wall carpeting, and you have a "home sweet home" for the accumulation of animal dander and dust mites.

Air pollution has become a fact of modern life. It is also a possible asthma trigger. Ozone, nitric oxide, acid aerosols, and diesel exhaust fumes can irritate the airways in people with asthma. Asthma investigators recently have found a strong correlation between ozone (smog) levels and serious asthma attacks. Some recent studies have indicated that air pollution, while acting as an asthma trigger, may also promote chronic airway inflammation and leave the airways more sensitive to ragweed. These studies have found that in addition to irritating the airways, ozone and diesel fumes may increase the number of IgE antibodies in the lungs of people with asthma. Doctors have found that exposure to ozone and diesel fumes increases a person's reactions to such allergens as ragweed and some fungi. This may cause people with asthma who have been repeatedly exposed to high levels of ozone and diesel fumes to be more likely to have allergic reactions to ragweed and fungi.

Children with asthma may be especially hard hit by the effects of air pollution. On days when pollution, such as the levels of ozone and exhaust particles, is particularly high, some hospitals have reported visits by and admissions of children with asthma to be 20 to 30 percent higher than normal.

Emotional reactions have been thought to cause asthma attacks for some time, but only recently have doctors begun to understand that while certain emotions can trigger an attack, asthma is not a psychological disease. Crying, laughing, yelling, and hyperventilating can trigger asthma attacks because the increased frequency and force of the air passing through the airways irritates the linings. Doctors are just beginning to understand that stress can trigger an attack because many of the chemicals released by the body in response to stress can also cause the airways to constrict. The effect of stress on asthma symptoms varies from one person to the next. It should be considered a factor in people who have difficult-to-control asthma symptoms and are under a great deal of stress.

PATIENT CHECKLIST

What You Should Avoid
- ❑ Active smoking
- ❑ Passive smoking
- ❑ Certain drugs used to treat high blood pressure and some heart conditions
- ❑ Aspirin and aspirin-related products

What You Should Reduce Your Exposure To If They Trigger Asthma Attacks
- ❑ Dust and dust mites
- ❑ Other common allergens such as cockroaches; pets; feather beds, pillows, and comforters; and pollens
- ❑ Food additives such as sulfites
- ❑ Indoor air pollution such as perfumes and smoke from wood-burning stoves

What You Should Not Avoid
- ❑ Normal social activities
- ❑ Most exercise
- ❑ Sports

Changes in the weather can trigger an asthma attack. Windy, rainy conditions can cause increased amounts of pollen to be washed from trees and grass and blown around in the air. When air gets stagnant or during a weather phenomenon known as a thermal inversion, the levels of air pollutants can climb dangerously high for people with asthma.

Medications, most commonly aspirin and beta blockers, can trigger asthma attacks. Up to one of every four adults with asthma is sensitive to aspirin and nonsteroidal anti-inflammatory drugs such as ibuprofen, contained in the pain medications Advil, Nuprin, and Motrin. It is less common for children with asthma to be aspirin-sensitive. It is not known how aspirin can trigger an asthma attack. The drug does not appear to stimulate the IgE antibodies and therefore is unlikely to be considered an allergen.

Beta blockers are drugs used to treat high blood pressure, heart disease, and the eye disorder glaucoma. Beta blockers can cause severe asthma attacks in people who are sensitive to them. They also may intensify allergic reactions to other substances. Other heart medications may cause similar reactions.

Doctors agree that people with asthma who are sensitive to aspirin or other medications should avoid these drugs. Other high blood pressure medications often can be safely substituted for beta blockers in people with asthma. And the drug acetaminophen, contained in the pain reliever Tylenol, rarely causes reactions in people with asthma who are sensitive to aspirin.

Sulfites are food additives that are used to prevent browning and discoloration of some foods. Children rarely are sensitive to sulfites, but ingestion of the chemicals can trigger an attack in some adults with severe asthma. Some of the more common foods and beverages that contain sulfites are avocados, certain baked products, beets and beet sugar, corn sweeteners, dried fruits, fresh shrimp, fruit drinks, gelatin, potatoes, fresh vegetables, wine, and cider.

4 / Treating Asthma in Adults

NOW THAT YOU UNDERSTAND WHAT CAN PREDISPOSE PEOPLE to develop asthma and what factors can promote and trigger an asthma attack, you are ready to learn how to take charge of this disease through the proper use of medications. Treating many diseases is a relatively simple process. For instance, if you have an infection, your doctor may prescribe an antibiotic that you must take at predetermined times of the day for a very well defined period of time.

That is not the case with asthma. Asthma medications must be tailored to the individual. Doctors determine how severe a case of asthma is before prescribing a medication or combination of medications. Some of these drugs are taken on a regular basis, while others are used only when an asthma sufferer has trouble breathing. You need to learn about these medications and about your own body. You must learn to identify the signs of an impending asthma attack so that you can use the proper combination of medications early in an attack to prevent it from becoming severe.

This means that in addition to learning about your asthma medications, you also must learn about the devices used to monitor when your asthma may be getting worse. By keeping a diary of your asthma symptoms and breathing function with a peak flow meter, you can predict when an asthma attack may be approaching. In this chapter you will learn about the different asthma medications available and how you can monitor your disease right from your own home or office.

A number of recent advances in the field of asthma have led to the development of new drugs to help control asthma. None of these developments is as important as the recognition that asthma can be controlled only through the regular use of drugs that reduce the underlying inflammation in the airways. We have learned that asthma is a chronic disease that causes the airways and lungs of sufferers to be habitually inflamed. When a person with asthma comes into contact with an asthma trigger, this chronic inflammation can cause an asthma attack. As little as 10 years ago, asthma medications were designed to be used only after a person started wheezing. Now doctors can prescribe from a host of newer medications that reduce the underlying airway inflammation and thus lower the number of wheezing attacks that people with asthma suffer.

"Sal"

Sal remembers his first asthma attack happening while he was on a navy freighter off the coast of Italy during the Second World War. "It wasn't even really an attack," Sal recalls. "It was more like a little tightness in my chest. We were on maneuvers and things were very busy. I was 17 years old and fit as an ox; it was the first time I had ever felt anything like that." But with the war to occupy him, the feeling passed and Sal didn't give it another thought — until he was back home about 20 years later.

"I was working as a plumber and we were installing the pipes for a new wing at a New York City hospital," Sal recalls. "I remember it had been raining for a few days and it was real cold and raw. The basement was flooded and very musty. The first thing that both the doctor and I thought was that I had caught a cold or flu." Sal remembers he had a scratchy feeling in his throat and was sneezing and sniffling. But more alarming was that for the first time since the war he felt tightness in his chest. He began wheezing, and instead of it getting any better he found that the wheezing, coughing, and shortness of breath just weren't going away.

Sal went back to the doctor because his breathing was getting even worse. "The doctor examined me and told me he thought I had asthma. I couldn't believe it. I mean, how could I develop asthma all of a sudden at almost 40 years old?" Sal learned that he is one of the many people with asthma who don't develop symptoms until later in life. The American Lung Association estimates that nearly 1.6 million Americans with asthma are age 65 or older. Once these people develop asthma as adults, many remember having had mild breathing problems as children, just like Sal.

In the 1960s, when Sal was having his first major bout with asthma, there wasn't much doctors could do to control his disease. "They told me that my breathing problems would flare up every once in a while and that there wasn't much I could do other than wait for that to happen." Once Sal's breathing problems did worsen, he had a liquid he was supposed to take to relax his constricted airways. If that didn't do the trick, Sal was off to the hospital for a shot of epinephrine and perhaps a course of oral steroids.

When Sal was first diagnosed with asthma, doctors did not understand the disease as they do today. Asthma was thought of as an episodic disease that occasionally flared up and needed to be treated. But as the years passed and doctors uncovered some of the mysteries surrounding asthma, they found that it is a chronic disease that causes the airways to be chronically inflamed and twitchy. This twitchiness can cause asthma attacks of wheezing when the person is exposed to some asthma trigger.

Today Sal is still working as a plumber, and at age 67 his asthma is almost completely controlled. Sal uses an inhaled steroid three times a day to reduce the underlying inflammation in his lungs and make it less likely that he will suffer an asthma attack. When an attack does strike, he uses an inhaled drug called metaproterenol to reverse the constriction in his airways. "I have not had to go to a hospital for my asthma or use oral steroids in years," Sal says. "My asthma is under control; it doesn't stop me from working or playing with my three grandchildren." None of Sal's two children or five grandchildren have shown any sign of asthma or allergies.

Sal was lucky that he was able to get the proper care for asthma at a time when less was known about the disease than now. But adults who develop asthma do not have to rely on luck anymore. Doctors can readily diagnose asthma in adults and have a variety of medications they can prescribe to reverse an asthma attack and prevent many from ever starting. ❏

The following paragraphs describe the categories of drugs your doctor can choose from when developing your personalized asthma maintenance program.

Beta-adrenergic drugs, also known as beta agonists, are adrenaline-like drugs used to relieve attacks of wheezing. They work by easing the constriction of the bronchial tubes brought on by exposure to asthma triggers. These drugs are excellent at providing temporary relief from an asthma attack, but they do not reduce the chronic inflammation in the lungs of people with asthma and therefore are usually only one of the drugs a person with moderate to severe asthma should take. They also may be used before exercise to limit exercise-induced asthma. There are some indications that newer, longer-acting beta-adrenergic drugs may act to prevent some asthma attacks and thus reduce the need for inhaled steroids.

Corticosteroids, which can be inhaled or taken in pill form, work by reducing the underlying chronic inflammation in the airways of people with asthma. Inhaled steroids do not relieve temporary attacks of wheezing and consequently are used with adrenergic drugs as part of an overall asthma treatment plan. Inhaled steroids now are considered essential in treating people with asthma who have moderate to severe symptoms. Short, 7- to 10-day treatments with oral steroids occasionally are used in people with asthma who have severe symptoms that are not being helped by other medications. Occasionally oral steroids may have to be used for prolonged periods in people with severe asthma.

Theophylline is an oral drug that is used to treat asthma flare-ups and to reduce chronic constriction of the bronchioles. Doctors often recommend that this drug be taken at night to reduce the frequency of nighttime asthma attacks.

Cromolyn and *nedocromil* are inhaled drugs that can prevent asthma attacks when taken before exercise or exposure to allergens. These drugs are more commonly used to reduce airway inflammation for long-term preventive asthma care in children. (For more about their use in children, see chapter 5.)

Closely following your doctor's instructions for taking asthma medications is essential for controlling the disease. Preventive asthma medications, such as inhaled steroids, must be taken regularly according to your doctor's advice. These medications work best when they are used on a continual basis, regardless of whether you are experiencing breathing problems. Inhaled adrenergic drugs, especially the new, longer-acting compounds, may be prescribed for regular use, or your doctor may suggest you use these medications only to reverse an asthma attack.

If after consulting with your doctor you still do not understand which medications should be used at different times during an asthma attack, it may be that you still do not understand how asthma and asthma medications work in the body, or your doctor may not have adequately explained your condition. In either case, you must press for a complete explanation. Do not be afraid to ask your doctor what you might consider "stupid questions." If you are to properly control asthma, you must have a full understanding of how severe your disease is and what medications can best treat it.

Before you leave the doctor's office, you should know:

- the name of the drug or drugs your doctor has prescribed and what these agents are supposed to do

- precisely how much medication you should take, and when and for how long these medications should be used

- the amount of time it takes for the medications to work

- what to expect regarding possible side effects

- what you should do if your asthma drug is not providing relief of your symptoms

- what you should do if you miss a dose or take an extra dose by mistake

- what to do if your symptoms worsen despite using your prescribed medications

Inhaled Beta-Adrenergic Drugs

As little as 10 years ago, most people with asthma who went to a hospital received an injection of epinephrine or adrenaline to reverse wheezing attacks. While the therapy was very effective in restoring breathing within minutes, it came with a number of side effects. These injections often caused jitteriness, restlessness, anxiety, headache, and a rapid or irregular heartbeat.

Today many doctors and emergency rooms give similar drugs in an aerosolized form through a compressor-driven nebulizer. Because the drug is inhaled directly into the lungs, it goes right to work on the bronchioles, reversing constriction and widening the airways. Consequently, a much lower dose can be used, and many of the side effects associated with epinephrine injections can be avoided. Nebulizers are available for regular home and emergency use and are a good way for parents to get inhaled asthma medications to their children's lungs.

Adrenergic drugs also are given in a metered-dose inhaler, a hand-held canister and mouthpiece that delivers a mist of the drug directly to the airways. Adrenergic drugs in a metered-dose inhaler have become standard therapy for most people with asthma. They are often used alone by people with mild or intermittent asthma, or in conjunction with anti-inflammatory medications by people with moderate or severe disease.

The only drawback to asthma drugs in metered-dose inhalers is learning how to use the devices. Even after people master the use of an inhaler, they often lapse back into bad habits when rushed. The proper use of a metered-dose inhaler is detailed later in this chapter.

Inhaled beta-adrenergic drugs are used by people with asthma because they:

- treat all levels of asthma attacks, from mild to moderate to severe
- quickly reverse constricted bronchioles, restoring breathing within minutes
- prevent bronchoconstriction from exercise, cold air, and other asthma triggers
- relieve sudden asthma attacks
- provide relief from wheezing during the time it takes for longer-acting drugs, such as theophylline, to work

Inhaled Adrenergic Drugs

Generic Name	Brand Names
albuterol	Proventil, Ventolin
bitolterol	Tornalate
metaproterenol	Alupent
isoetharine	Bronkometer, Bronkosol
isoproterenol	Isuprel
pirbuterol	Maxair
salmeterol	Serevent
terbutaline	Brethaire, Brethine

Effects: Inhaled adrenergic drugs relax the constricted muscles encircling the airways and thus open tightened airways during an asthma attack.

Possible side effects: Increased heart rate, palpitations, chest tightness, nervousness, sleeplessness, headache, nausea, vomiting, tremors, or shakiness. An increased heart rate or chest pain resulting from use of inhaled adrenergic drugs should be discussed with your doctor.

Time considerations: Inhaled adrenergic drugs begin working to open the airways in about 5 minutes or less. Their effects last for 4 to 6 hours. Salmeterol, or Serevent, is a new beta-adrenergic drug. Unlike other inhaled adrenergic drugs, salmeterol does not immediately relieve asthma attacks. It works to prevent the muscles surrounding the airways from becoming constricted. The drug's effects last for 12 hours.

Doses: Two puffs of the inhaler given over 2 minutes when needed to control wheezing. This dosage may be repeated several times a day as determined by your doctor. Do not increase this dose if you still are wheezing after using your inhaled adrenergic drug. Persistent symptoms after using an inhaled adrenergic drug may mean that the underlying inflammation in your airways is too severe and must be reduced with other medications. People with mild or intermittent asthma use their inhaled adrenergic drugs only when they feel an attack of wheezing coming on. However, you still should be careful not to exceed the maximum daily dose.

Comments: These drugs may be used about 15 minutes before exercising by people with exercise-induced asthma. Proper use of the inhaler is critical when using these agents.

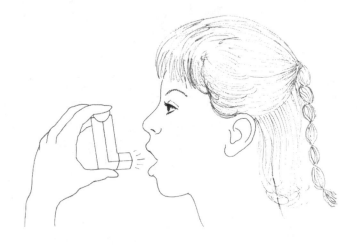

By learning how to properly use a metered-dose inhaler, people with asthma can reverse most attacks.

Instructions for Using a Metered-Dose Inhaler

- Sit comfortably and hold head upright or tilted slightly backward.
- Shake the inhaler very well immediately before each use. Remove the cap from the mouthpiece.
- Exhale completely.

- Open mouth wide and hold mouthpiece about 1 to 2 inches from your mouth. Do not put the mouthpiece in your mouth unless you are using a spacer—a tubelike device that attaches to the mouthpiece and collects the medication mist for easy inhalation. (Spacers are discussed in detail in chapter 5.)

- With the mouth open, take in a slow, deep breath through the mouth and at the same time firmly press down on the canister to discharge the medication.

- Hold breath for 5 to 10 seconds and move the inhaler away from your mouth.

- Breathe out slowly.

- Wait from 2 to 5 minutes before repeating this routine for a second puff.

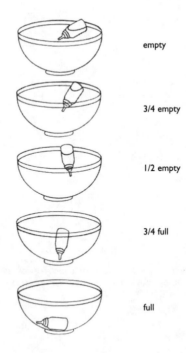

empty

3/4 empty

1/2 empty

3/4 full

full

Regularly check your metered-dose inhaler to determine how much medication is left.

Additional Tips for Using an Inhaler

- Always shake the canister well before each use.

- Use only as often as directed by your doctor. The usual dose of inhaled adrenergic drugs is two puffs only when needed to control wheezing. See your doctor if you are still experiencing symptoms, but do not increase the dose on your own.

- Ask your doctor about using an inhaled adrenergic drug to open your airways before using a cromolyn or steroid inhaler.

- Ask your doctor about using an inhaled adrenergic drug about 15 minutes before exercising if you suffer from exercise-induced asthma.

- Always keep the protective cap on the inhaler when it is not in use.

- Replace your inhaler when the canister is one-fourth full. Place the canister in a bowl of water and use the illustration on page 40 to test how much medication remains in the container.

It takes time and practice to master the use of an asthma inhaler. But with repeated use, you will become very adept at getting these needed drugs directly to your lungs. Some common mistakes when using an inhaler include:

- *Inhaling too fast,* causing much of the drug to be deposited in your mouth or throat, so that it never makes it to your lungs

- *Holding your breath for less than 10 seconds* and not allowing the medication to settle before being exhaled from the bronchioles

- *Not waiting long enough before a second inhalation* and inhaling the drug through still-constricted airways

- *Forgoing a second inhalation* and not delivering enough medication to your airways

- *Not using a spacer* to help deliver the medication mist to the lungs, especially in the young and elderly

Oral Adrenergic Drugs

Oral adrenergic drugs may be used for some people with asthma who are not getting adequate relief from inhaled agents. These drugs ease constriction of the airways but do not work as quickly as the inhaled versions. Some of these drugs provide long-term relief of bronchospasm and can prevent nighttime asthma attacks.

Oral Adrenergic Drugs

Generic Name	Brand Names
albuterol	Proventil, Ventolin
metaproterenol	Alupent
terbutaline	Brethine

Effects: Oral adrenergic drugs relax the constricted muscles surrounding the bronchioles, allowing them to open more completely.

Possible side effects: Similar to those of inhaled adrenergic agents and can include increased heart rate, palpitations, chest pain, nervousness, sleeplessness, headache, nausea, vomiting, tremors, or shakiness.

Time considerations: These drugs usually take effect within about 30 minutes and last for 6 to 8 hours.

Doses: The dose of oral adrenergic drugs varies greatly and is determined by the type of drug used, the patient's weight, and how often and severely the patient is experiencing attacks. They typically are taken every 6 to 8 hours, with the final dose of pills a few hours before bedtime. Liquid versions of some oral adrenergic drugs are available and are primarily used for children. (Liquid adrenergic drugs are discussed further in chapter 5.)

Comments: Oral adrenergic drugs typically are reserved for people with asthma who cannot use inhaled adrenergic agents. The drugs may also be used to prevent nighttime wheezing attacks.

Inhaled Steroids

The development of inhaled steroids has been an important advance in the treatment of asthma. Steroids are among the few medications available to reverse the underlying inflammation of the airways in people with asthma. It is only by reversing this underlying inflammation that many asthma attacks can be prevented. Doctors working on the federal government's National Asthma Education and

Prevention Program have recommended that inhaled steroids be used by virtually all people who have moderate or severe asthma. People with moderate to severe asthma often are given both an inhaled steroid to reduce airway inflammation and an inhaled adrenergic drug to reverse any breakthrough asthma attacks.

Inhaled Steroids

Generic Name	Brand Names
beclomethasone dipropionate	Beclovent, Vanceril
flunisolide	Aerobid
triamcinolone acetonide	Azmacort

Steroid pills for oral use have been available for years, but oral steroids taken for prolonged periods (several weeks or more) can cause numerous side effects and are not recommended for chronic use. Inhaled steroids deliver the drug directly to the lungs. Consequently, much lower doses can be used to reduce airway inflammation, thus avoiding many side effects. Numerous studies have shown inhaled steroids to be safe even when used for long-term asthma control. The most serious side effect from inhaled steroids is the development of an oral infection called thrush. This infection can produce creamy white patches in the mouth and must be treated with oral anti-infective drugs. Most people can avoid mouth infections by properly gargling and rinsing the mouth after each use of the steroid inhaler. Devices called spacers, which are attached to the mouthpieces of asthma inhalers, also may reduce the chance of developing mouth infections. Spacers collect the mist from an inhaler in a large tube before it is inhaled, thus reducing the amount of medication that settles in the mouth. (More information about spacers can be found in chapter 5.)

Effects: Inhaled steroids reduce the underlying inflammation in the airways of people with asthma, making it less likely that they will experience an asthma attack when exposed to some asthma promoter or trigger.

Possible side effects: Mouth infections, resulting in creamy white, curdlike patches in the mouth, are the most common side effect. Other, less severe side effects that tend to go away after repeated use of a steroid inhaler include cough, hoarseness, throat irritation, and dry mouth. It is very important that you gargle and rinse your mouth after each puff of a steroid inhaler to reduce the chances of developing these side effects.

Time considerations: Inhaled steroids do not relieve asthma attacks. These drugs work slowly to reduce inflammation in the airways, thus preventing many attacks from occurring. It may take from 2 to 4 weeks of regular use before inhaled steroids can exert their maximum anti-inflammatory effect.

Doses: The dose of inhaled steroids depends on how severe your asthma is and what type of steroid your doctor prescribes. Doses range from 2 puffs taken 2 to 4 times a day. Steroid inhalers must be used regularly to be effective. This means that even though you may not be experiencing trouble breathing, you must continue to use your steroid inhaler as recommended by your doctor.

Comments: Many people with asthma use inhaled steroids for long periods of time. Regular use of these drugs reduces airway inflammation and the chance that you will suffer an asthma attack. These medications do not relieve asthma attacks but should be used regularly, even when you are wheezing.

Important Information and Tips for Taking Inhaled Steroids

- Using a spacer can improve delivery of this medication to your lungs and may reduce possible steroid side effects.

- Remember, inhaled steroids do not relieve asthma attacks.

- Follow your doctor's advice for using these drugs. Inhaled steroids must be used regularly to reduce airway inflammation. It may take from 2 to 4 weeks before you notice full effects. Continue taking them even when you are not having trouble breathing. Do not increase, decrease, or stop using these inhalers on your own.

- If you miss a dose of this drug, use it as soon as possible.

- If you develop signs of a mouth infection, a sore mouth, or a rash, see your doctor; do not stop using the inhaler unless instructed to do so. If your asthma symptoms do not improve after 4 weeks, see your doctor.

- Always gargle and rinse your mouth with water after using the inhaler to reduce the chance of developing a mouth infection or mouth irritation.

- Tell your doctor or dentist that you are using these medications before having any surgery, immunizations, dental work, or emergency treatments.

Oral Steroids

People with asthma who are having significant trouble breathing and are not being adequately helped by other asthma medications may receive short courses of oral steroid pills. Treatment with oral steroids is often called pulse or burst treatment because it is given in relatively high doses for short periods of time. Oral steroids are very effective in reducing the underlying inflammation in the airways. Doctors often give oral steroids to reduce airway inflammation in people with asthma who are having significant trouble breathing. The drugs are ordinarily stopped after a few days, and inhaled steroids are then used to continue to reduce inflammation. Because of their potential side effects, oral steroids should not be used on a continuous basis except in severe cases.

Oral Steroids

Generic Name	Brand Names
dexamethasone	Decadron
hydrocortisone	Hydrocortone
methylprednisolone	Medrol Tablets
prednisone	Prednisone

Effects: Oral steroids reverse airway inflammation and are used to ease the severity of severe asthma attacks.

Possible side effects: Prolonged use of oral steroids can cause severe side effects that should be reported to your doctor. Those side effects include decreased or blurred vision, frequent urination, increased thirst, mood changes, or skin rash. Less severe side effects include increase in appetite, weight gain, insomnia, nervousness, stomach upset, and restlessness. Very long-term use increases the risk of developing cataracts, ulcers, and susceptibility to bone fractures, though very few people with asthma need long-term oral steroid therapy.

Time considerations: Oral steroids begin to take effect within 6 hours and reach their peak about 12 hours after being taken.

Doses: Doses of oral steroids vary with the type of drug used, the patient's weight, and the severity of the asthma. A typical burst course of oral steroids might be 30 to 60 mg of prednisone once a day for 7 to 10 days. A recent study by researchers in Denver suggests that when prescribed to prevent severe nighttime asthma attacks, oral steroids may be most effective when taken at about 3 P.M. A midafternoon dose of oral steroids was more effective in reducing nighttime airway inflammation than a dose taken at either 8 A.M. or 8 P.M.

Comments: Oral steroids are very effective for people with severe asthma symptoms who are not being helped by other asthma medications. Oral steroids control and prevent airway inflammation and may get people with severe asthma back under control so that other asthma medications can better manage their disease. They should not be used for long periods of time except in severe cases.

Important Information and Tips for Taking Oral Steroids

- Take exactly as instructed by your doctor.
- Take with milk, food, or antacids to reduce stomach problems (as prescribed by your doctor).
- Aspirin may worsen the stomach problems associated with oral steroids.
- Tell your doctor or dentist you are using this drug before having any treatment, dental work, surgery, or emergency treatment, or if you have a serious infection or injury.
- If you miss a dose and your normal schedule is one dose every other day, take it as soon as you remember; if it is in the same morning, then continue your normal schedule. If you do not remember until the afternoon, wait and take it the following morning; then skip a day and resume your normal schedule. If you miss a dose and your normal schedule is one dose a day, take it as soon as you remember and continue with your regular schedule; if you miss an entire day, skip that dose.
- Never decrease, skip, or stop taking steroids on your own.
- Call your doctor or nurse if you have any increase in signs of infection or illness, including fever or runny nose. Steroids can mask signs of infection.

Theophylline

Theophylline and theophylline-like drugs are useful in treating mild to moderate asthma attacks, as well as in preventing attacks, when used on a daily basis. The drugs often are used in combination with other asthma medications. Many of these compounds, which come in pill form, are in slow- or timed-release preparations. Many people with asthma find these drugs convenient because they are taken only once or twice a day.

Theophylline and Theophylline-like Drugs

Generic Name	Brand Names
aminophylline	Aminophylline tablets
theophylline	Aerolate, Quibron, Respbid, Slo-bid, Slo-Phyllin, Theochron, Theo-Dur, Theolair, Uniphyl Tablets

Theophylline belongs to a group of chemicals called the xanthines. Its chemical structure is similar to that of caffeine, but its effects on various body systems are much more intense. This group of chemicals has effects on various parts of the body, including the nervous system and the brain, the muscles, the heart, the kidneys, and the stomach. There are many factors that affect the way theophylline acts within the body; these factors include the rate at which the body absorbs theophylline, the time it takes to metabolize, or eliminate, the drug, and the extent to which theophylline is distributed throughout the body.

Much has been written about the possible side effects of theophylline, especially in children. (The effects of theophylline in children are discussed in chapter 5.) In adults, many factors can affect how quickly theophylline is eliminated from the body. Various foods and medications can slow or speed the process by which the body gets rid of the drug. If this process is slowed, excess amounts of theophylline may build up in the body, leading to possible side effects; conversely, if the process is speeded up, people with asthma may not get adequate amounts of the drug in their blood. This may hamper the ability of theophylline to relieve bronchoconstriction.

Certain drugs, such as erythromycin and other antibiotics, as well as the ulcer medication cimetidine, may interfere with the body's ability to get rid of theophylline. Some respiratory infections may have the same effect, causing theophylline levels to become dangerously high. Other factors, such as smoke, charcoal-broiled foods, meals high in protein, and the seizure medications phenobarbital and phenytonin, also called Dilantin, can speed up the rate at which the body eliminates theophylline. In these cases, theophylline levels can become too low to be of benefit.

Even without the effect of certain medications, viruses, and foods, theophylline levels vary throughout the day and night. Newer, slow-release theophylline preparations reduce much of this fluctuation but still require that you take theophylline pills at the times your doctor has recommended.

Effects: Theophylline relaxes the muscles surrounding the airway tree, allowing the airways to open more completely.

Possible side effects: Stomach upset, nausea and vomiting, restlessness, rapid heart rate, wakefulness, irritability, dizziness, and palpitations. The side effects of theophylline are most common within the first few days of starting therapy. These side effects may be avoided by starting at a low dose and working up to the dose needed to reduce airway constriction. Some slow-release preparations, which distribute theophylline more evenly, may result in fewer side effects.

Time considerations: Slow-release theophylline preparations can be taken every 12 or 24 hours, regular theophylline preparations as often as every 8 hours. They typically begin to work about 1 to 2 hours after being taken and reach a maximum effective level in the body about 2 to 6 hours after the second dose is taken, or about 14 to 18 hours after the very first dose. Liquid preparations typically given to children tend to act more quickly and last for shorter periods of time.

If you miss a dose and your schedule is to take one pill every 24 hours, take the missed dose when you remember if it is within 12 hours of the scheduled time, and then return to your normal schedule. If you remember 12 to 20 hours after the scheduled dose, take one-half of the dose and return to your regular schedule. If you remember after 20 hours from the missed dose, skip it and go on to the next dose.

If you miss a dose of theophylline and your schedule is to take one pill every 12 hours, take the missed dose when you remember, if it is within 2 hours of the scheduled time. If you remember within 8 hours of the scheduled dose, take the missed dose, take your next dose 2 hours later than usual, and then return to your regular schedule. If you don't remember to take the dose until more than 8 hours after the scheduled dose, take the missed dose and omit the next scheduled dose, then return to your normal schedule.

If you are taking a theophylline preparation that is scheduled for every 8 hours and you miss a dose for less than 6 hours, take the missed dose and space out the remaining doses of the day evenly. If you wait longer than 6 hours, omit the missed dose and go back to your regular schedule.

Doses: Determining the correct dose of theophylline is a complicated process that depends on how severe your asthma is, how much you weigh, and how sensitive you are to the drug. Your doctor will determine how much theophylline you need by taking blood samples. To reduce the rate of side effects from this drug, your doctor may use a slow-release version of the drug, which enters the body slowly and more evenly than traditional theophylline pills. If you are unable to take a slow-release theophylline pill, your doctor may attempt to reduce the side effects of theophylline by starting you on very low doses of the drug and gradually increasing these doses until you are taking a suitable amount.

Comments: Theophylline and theophylline-like drugs may be used by people with asthma symptoms who are not getting adequate relief of bronchoconstriction from inhaled or oral adrenergic drugs. Theophylline often is used in addition to adrenergic drugs to achieve the maximum possible relief of airway constriction.

Important Information and Tips for Taking Theophylline

- Theophylline must be taken regularly and spaced evenly over a 24-hour period. It usually takes 2 to 3 days for the medication to reach the ideal level in your blood.

- The medication reaches the bloodstream more quickly when taken on an empty stomach but may cause stomach upset.

- Take with a full glass of water.

- Do not increase the dose or frequency because it could cause serious side effects.

- Avoid large amounts of coffee, tea, colas, cocoa, and chocolate, as these foods and drinks may add to the stimulant effect of the medication.

- Your doctor may find it helpful to periodically monitor the amount of theophylline in your blood. Do not miss these appointments for blood work.

- Theophylline may react differently when you have a viral infection, smoke, eat charcoal-broiled foods, or take certain other medications, even if you are following your doctor's advice.

Cromolyn and Nedocromil

Cromolyn is an inhaled drug that may reduce the number of asthma attacks by blocking the release of chemicals that can trigger an attack. It is sold under the brand name Intal. This drug does not reduce wheezing and is of no help during an asthma attack. A new product called nedocromil, sold under the brand name Tilade, is often used as an anti-inflammatory drug in children with asthma and in adults who cannot tolerate inhaled steroids.

Effects: Cromolyn may reduce the number of asthma attacks and prevent exercise-induced asthma attacks and attacks triggered by allergens. Nedocromil may reduce the underlying inflammation in the airways of people with asthma.

Possible side effects: Generally few, but can include coughing, wheezing, and shortness of breath. Tilade may have a bad taste.

Time considerations: These drugs work to prevent some asthma attacks after about 4 weeks of use. Cromolyn should be used about 15 minutes before exposure to a known allergen (like cats or dogs) and a few minutes before exercise. Nedocromil is taken regularly to reduce airway inflammation.

Doses: Usually 2 puffs 4 times a day or (for cromolyn) as a treatment before exposure to allergens or exercise.

Comments: Cromolyn and nedocromil do not work in all people with asthma. For those in whom they do work, they are very safe and may control allergen- and exercise-induced asthma attacks, as well as reduce airway inflammation (in the case of nedocromil).

Other Drugs

Other drugs are generally given to control symptoms related to asthma or conditions that frequently occur in people with asthma. These include antibiotics to treat sinus infections and antihistamines to control allergies. (More information about these drugs appears in chapter 8.)

THE FUTURE IS NOW FOR ASTHMA MEDICATIONS

New drugs that may help "mop up" or block the chemicals that can cause your airways to become inflamed and irritated are now available. The drugs, called leukotriene inhibitors, may help turn off asthma attacks before they ever start by blocking the activity of chemicals called leukotrienes. These are one of the many irritating substances released by mast cells after you are exposed to an allergen or asthma trigger. Because the drugs are so new there are no government-approved recommendations on where they fit into the treatment plan for people with asthma. The first of these drugs to be approved by the U.S. Food and Drug Administration in 1996, zafirlukast (sold under the brand name Accolate), must be taken twice a day in pill form for the prevention of asthma in people aged 12 and older. Because the drug works to prevent asthma attacks, it does not help reverse bouts of wheezing once they occur. A second leukotriene inhibitor, zileuton (sold under the brand name Zyflo), was approved at the end of 1996. These drugs are the first two in what promises to be a long line of new asthma medications that may help turn off asthma attacks before they ever start.

A Step-by-Step Approach to Treating Asthma

New guidelines published by the federal government's National Asthma Education and Prevention Program in 1997 classify asthma in four degrees of severity: mild intermittent, mild persistent, moderate persistent, and severe persistent. The guidelines include a suggested step-by-step approach to treating the different classes of asthma severity.

Mild Intermittent Asthma

Characterized by symptoms two or fewer times a week, two or fewer episodes of nighttime asthma symptoms per month, and lung function at 80 percent of normal or greater. Asthma flare-ups are brief (from a few hours to a few days); intensity may vary.

Daily Medication: No daily medication is needed.

Quick Relief: Inhaled beta$_2$-agonists as needed for symptoms.

Mild Persistent Asthma

Characterized by symptoms more than twice a week but less than once every day; nighttime symptoms more than twice a month, and lung function at 80 percent of normal or greater. Asthma flare-ups may affect activity.

Daily Medication: Either low doses of inhaled corticosteroid, or cromolyn or nedocromil. Sustained-release theophylline is an alternative. Zafirlukast or zileuton may also be considered for patients 12 years of age or older.

Quick Relief: Inhaled beta$_2$-agonists as needed for symptoms.

Moderate Persistent Asthma

Characterized by daily symptoms and daily use of inhaled short-acting beta$_2$-agonists; nighttime symptoms more than once a week, and lung function at 60 percent to 80 percent of normal. Asthma flare-ups affect activity; they occur two or more times a week and may last days.

Daily Medication: Either inhaled corticosteroid (medium dose) or inhaled corticosteroid (low–medium dose) and a long-acting bronchodilator, especially for nighttime symptoms: either long-acting beta$_2$-agonists, sustained-release theophylline, or long-acting beta$_2$-agonist tablets. If needed: anti-inflammatory inhaled corticosteroids (medium–high dose) AND long-acting bronchodilator, especially for nighttime symptoms: either long-acting inhaled beta$_2$-agonists, sustained-release theophylline, or long-acting beta$_2$-agonist tablets.

Quick Relief: Inhaled beta$_2$-agonists as needed for symptoms.

Severe Persistent Asthma

Characterized by continual symptoms, limited physical activity, and frequent asthma flare-ups; frequent nighttime symptoms; and lung function at 60 percent of normal or less.

Daily Medication: Inhaled corticosteroid (high dose) and either long-acting inhaled beta$_2$-agonists, sustained-release theophylline, or long-acting beta$_2$-agonist tablets AND corticosteroid tablets or syrup long term.

Quick Relief: Inhaled beta$_2$-agonists as needed for symptoms.

Peak Flow Meters

Asthma attacks do not start without warning. They often begin with a feeling of chest tightness, coughing, and wheezing. A peak flow meter may help you spot the signs of an asthma attack even before they lead to these symptoms. By regularly monitoring the condition of your airways, you will be better able to predict when an asthma attack may strike. This is important because early use of inhaled adrenergic drugs can lessen the severity of asthma attacks. Regular monitoring may also help identify times when your airways are becoming so inflamed and blocked that your doctor may need to prescribe new medications to reverse the inflammation before it leads to a severe bout of wheezing. You can regularly monitor your airway function at home with a portable device called a peak flow meter.

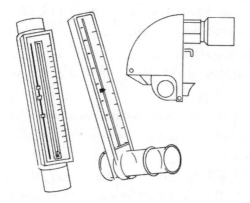

Peak flow meters can help predict when an asthma attack might strike.

What Is a Peak Flow Meter?

A peak flow meter is a portable, inexpensive, hand-held device used to measure how air flows from your lungs in one "fast blast"—in other words, your ability to push air out of your lungs. Since one of the signs of an impending asthma attack is a reduced ability to push air out of your lungs, a peak flow meter can help predict when an asthma attack may be approaching.

Peak flow meters are available in two ranges: low-range meters are generally used for small children; standard meters are used for older children, teenagers, and adults. Several types of peak flow meters are available. Talk to your doctor or pharmacist about which meter to use.

Not all doctors use a peak flow meter when managing children and adults with asthma. Many doctors believe that a peak flow meter may be of most use to people with moderate to severe asthma. If your asthma is mild, or if you do not use daily medications, a peak flow meter may not be necessary.

How to Use a Peak Flow Meter

Step 1: Before each use, make sure the sliding marker or arrow on the peak flow meter is at the bottom of the numbered scale.

Step 2: Stand up straight. Empty your mouth of any food or gum. Take as deep a breath as you can, put the mouthpiece of the meter in your mouth, and tightly close your lips around the mouthpiece. Be sure to keep your tongue away from the opening in the mouthpiece. Blow out as hard and as quickly as you can until you have emptied nearly all the air from your lungs.

Step 3: The force of the air coming from your lungs causes the marker or arrow on the meter to move up the numbered scale. Note this number.

Step 4: Repeat the entire routine three times. You know you have done the routine correctly when all three readings are very close together.

Step 5: Record the highest of the three readings; do not take an average of the three. You can't breathe out too much when using your peak flow meter, but you can breathe out too little or too slowly. You want to record the highest number (your best attempt).

Step 6: Measure your peak flow rate close to the same time each day. Talk to your doctor about the best times to measure your peak flow. One suggestion is to measure your peak flow rate upon arising in the morning and again in the early evening. You may want to measure your peak flow before and after using your asthma medications to get a sense of how much improvement in airway function your medications give you. Just make sure to do it the same way and at the same times each day.

Step 7: Keep a chart of your peak flow rate and discuss it with your doctor. There is a sample peak flow chart in this chapter.

What Is a Normal Peak Flow Rate?

A normal peak flow rate is based on a person's age, height, sex, and race. A standardized normal may be obtained from charts comparing you to people who do not have breathing problems. You and your doctor should discuss what peak flow rate is normal for you.

How Can I Determine a Normal Peak Flow Rate for Me?

After using a peak flow meter for a few days when you are not experiencing asthma symptoms, you will be able to see what your best peak flow rate is. Peak flow meters measure lung function in the amount of liters of air you can force from your lungs per minute. Once you have determined what your best peak flow rate is when you are not experiencing asthma symptoms, you will be able to use a handy three-color guide to tell you when you may be on the verge of an asthma attack.

The green, or OK, zone: When your peak flow is in the green zone, your lungs are operating at between 80 and 100 percent of your best peak flow rate. A reading in this zone means that your asthma is under reasonable control. Exposure to a mild asthma trigger may not cause any breathing problems. If asthma symptoms do occur, they generally come on gradually, giving adequate notice to begin treatment. You should continue to take whatever asthma medications are prescribed. If you have mild asthma, this may mean no treatment at all.

The yellow, or caution, zone: When your peak flow is in the yellow zone, it means that your lungs are operating at between 50 and 80 percent of your best rate. It is time for you to make decisions about controlling your asthma before it gets out of hand. A yellow-zone reading means that your airways are narrowing and may require additional treatment. Exposure to a minor asthma trigger may cause noticeable wheezing, while exposure to several triggers (for example, tobacco smoke on top of a respiratory infection) may produce significant breathing problems. Two peak flow readings in the yellow zone within 48 hours indicates you probably need additional medication and should call your doctor.

The red, or danger, zone: If your peak flow readings are in the red zone, your lungs are operating at less than 50 percent of their capacity. This means that your airways already have narrowed and are restricting your breathing. You should contact your doctor immediately.

My Peak Flow Rates

Name _____ Week Begining (Date) _____

Peak Flow Zones: Green Zone _____ Yellow Zone _____ Red Zone _____

Prescribed Medications (include dose and frequency) _____

Peak Flow Recording Times: _____ AM _____ PM

Day	Sunday		Monday		Tuesday		Wednesday		Thursday		Friday		Saturday	
Time	AM	PM	AM	PM	AM	PM	AM	PM	AM	PM	AM	PM	AM	PM
600														
550														
500														
450														
400														
350														
300														
250														
200														
150														
100														
Changes in Medicine														
Notes														

Your Peak Flow Rates (liters/minute)

An Asthma Emergency Plan

Now that you know what medications to take for your asthma and how to monitor your breathing with a peak flow meter, you can control and prevent many asthma attacks. But an attack still can happen even to people with asthma who are properly controlling their disease. It is a good idea to develop a plan for what to do during different phases of asthma. It takes the guesswork out of treating your asthma, and if you experience a severe asthma attack, an emergency plan will save valuable time. It also helps you to plan ahead, since you may not be thinking clearly once a severe asthma attack strikes.

You should talk to your doctor about developing a plan to manage your asthma through different phases of the disease. One way to do that is to base the plan on your peak flow readings. You can use the asthma plan in this chapter when you discuss devising your own asthma management plan with your doctor. Make sure you ask your doctor about what steps to take if your peak flow measurements enter the red zone. This is the danger area, and you should have a ready-to-use, mapped-out plan of what action to take.

The asthma management plan you develop with your doctor may have you maintain your normal asthma medications as long as your peak flow readings are in the green zone. Your doctor may want you to add a special medication or call for assistance if your peak flow readings fall into the yellow zone. Most important, your plan will prepare you to know when to go to the hospital or emergency room if your peak flow readings fall within the red zone. While this is unlikely to happen if you closely follow the advice of your doctor, a well-laid-out asthma management plan is just one more of the steps you need to take to control and live with this disease.

My Asthma Management Plan Based on Peak Flow Readings

Green Zone:_____To _____
I feel good—my plan is: _____
_____
_____
_____
_____
_____

Yellow Zone: _____To _____
I have some problems—my plan is: _____
_____
_____
_____
_____

Red Zone: below _____
I am not feeling well at all and am having problems
frequently—my plan is: _____
_____
_____
_____
_____

5 / Treating Asthma in Children

TREATING AND CONTROLLING ASTHMA IN CHILDREN IS A MATTER of partnerships. There is the relationship between the parents and the child with asthma, between the child and his or her doctor, and between the parents and the doctor. Parents are an important factor in the proper control of asthma in their children. If your child is to learn to live with and control this disease, you will need to become actively involved in his or her asthma care program. With the advice of your child's doctor, you can help tailor an asthma care program that is suited to your child's activities. You can also help educate your child about the signs of an impending asthma attack, the best times and ways to take asthma medications, and possible asthma promoters and triggers that can worsen your child's breathing.

Parents of very young children with asthma need to become keenly aware and observant of their children's symptoms. The children are often too young or inexperienced to recognize the signs of an impending asthma attack. As parents, you need to learn to recognize these signs in your children so that you can intervene early in the course of an asthma attack with medications to arrest and reverse airway constriction and inflammation. While many recommendations for asthma therapy exist, there is great room for individualizing asthma treatment, both in the types of medications used and the times and frequencies with which these medications are employed. By talking with your doctor and providing information on how your child responds to drugs, you can play an active role in deciding which medications may be best for your child and what medication schedules will be most successfully adhered to.

Parents are the principal administrators of medication for children with asthma. Very young children often are unable to master the intricacies involved in taking asthma medications. As parents, you can draw on a host of medication delivery devices to help your child get needed medications.

As your child with asthma grows older, you will find that he or she takes over many of these roles. Your child will learn to recognize when an attack of wheezing is approaching and will learn to use asthma inhalers and peak flow meters independently. And your child will become more familiar with the asthma promoters and triggers that can trip an attack and learn how to reduce his or her exposure to them. But *your* role in the partnership of asthma management in your children will remain. Children with asthma are no different from children who do not suffer from this disease. They play with other children, go to school, and take part in outside activities. And they are just as prone to the struggles of a child's daily routine and to the influences of peer pressure and group acceptance as are other children.

As parents, you should consider these factors when talking to your doctor about designing an asthma care program for your child. You will find that there is considerable flexibility. While some of this flexibility is at the doctor's discretion and concerns what medications are most appropriate for your child's symptoms and degree of asthma, much of this flexibility will be based on the child's level of activity and his or her comfort level in taking medications at different times during the day.

Many factors go into determining your child's asthma management plan. Your child may participate in sports or other outdoor activities. If this is the case, asthma medications that tend to reduce the chance of developing exercise-induced wheezing should be scheduled at times when they can exert their maximum effects. You also may find that your child with asthma is reluctant to take medications during the day at school. Or your child may simply forget to take these medications when faced with the normal school-day schedule. If these factors are at play in the management of your child's asthma, you should discuss them with your doctor. Properly controlled asthma depends on regularly following an asthma treatment plan. If your child is missing or skipping doses of medications, a new plan should be designed that is better suited to him or her. You and your doctor may decide that it is best that your child take the asthma medications before leaving for school and upon returning home. Typically, many asthma medications are given four times a day. However, it is possible to style an asthma management plan in which double doses of drugs are given only twice a day. This may not be the most ideal asthma management plan, but sometimes a good program that is followed is better than an ideal program that is ignored.

The most important point about treating asthma in children is the same as the most important factor in treating asthma in adults. Your child, just like an adult with asthma, needs medications to control the underlying inflammation in his or her airways. This is the case with all children who have moderate to severe asthma symptoms. If your child has very mild symptoms or experiences asthma attacks only infrequently, he or she may only require medications that quickly reverse these attacks. However, even children with mild asthma can often benefit from medications that may prevent asthma attacks brought on by exercise or exposure to allergens.

Many of the medications used to treat asthma in adults are also used in children with asthma. But there are some important differences. Doses of asthma medications for children, especially those taken by mouth, often are lower than those given to adults. This is primarily to minimize possible side effects. Asthma medications for children also may come in different forms. Adrenergic drugs, cromolyn, and nedocromil are all available in liquids that can be used in air-compressor delivery devices called nebulizers, and capsules containing a dry powder form of the drug can be inhaled directly into the lungs with a special inhaler. Adrenergic drugs are also available in pills or liquids to be taken by mouth.

Children with asthma may need special delivery systems to get asthma medications to their lungs. Very young children may need to have their medications delivered through a nebulizer or through a metered-dose inhaler with a spacer and face mask attached. Once children learn how to work a metered-dose inhaler on their own, a spacer is a good idea. Spacers are tubes that are attached to the end of a metered-dose inhaler and collect the medication mist before it is inhaled. They can make it easier for a child to coordinate using a metered-dose inhaler and may reduce the rate of side effects from some medications by cutting down on the amount of the drug that is deposited in the mouth. In this chapter you will learn about special considerations when giving asthma medications to children and about devices that can help get these medications to your child's lungs. (For a description of how to use peak flow meters, see chapter 4.)

Delivery Mechanisms

It's often difficult for children to master using a metered-dose inhaler. Unfortunately, medications delivered by these devices are the primary method of asthma treatment. Metered-dose inhalers require consid-

"Jessica"

Jessica was 18 months old when she was diagnosed as having asthma. Her parents remember the first attack starting with a common cold that kept getting worse, eventually affecting her breathing. They took Jessica to the hospital, where she was given an injection of epinephrine and some theophylline pills to take by mouth. Her breathing cleared up, but the pediatrician in the emergency room told her parents for the first time that Jessica had asthma. The doctor explained that she would probably grow out of her condition, but in the meantime they should be prepared to live through a number of similar asthma attacks. "We just didn't understand," remembers Jessica's mom, Mary. "We had never known anyone who had asthma and we didn't know what to expect. We were frightened for Jessica, and we weren't sure how this disease would affect her from here on in. The pediatrician told us to be on the lookout for signs of an attack and bring her back to the hospital when she had trouble breathing." While the treatment Jessica received on that first emergency room visit cleared up her breathing, and the theophylline pills kept her airways open for a while, about two weeks later she started wheezing and coughing all over again. "That's when I knew that this was something serious and that it was going to change all our lives," Mary says.

So Jessica's parents did what they were told. They watched for signs of wheezing and coughing in their daughter, and they rushed her to the emergency room whenever these signs of asthma flared, usually in the middle of the night. Most times, another injection of epinephrine cleared up her breathing problems, but occasionally she had to stay in the hospital overnight. "There were two times when her asthma was so severe that we had to leave her there, and that is one of the hardest things in the world to do," Mary says. "But they kept telling us that she would grow out of this, so we kept our fingers crossed and waited."

This pattern repeated itself for about three years. Jessica would have occasional nighttime asthma attacks, sometimes requiring a trip to the hospital, sometimes clearing up with medication. Severe asthma attacks struck, it seemed, every time Jessica caught a cold or flu. Jessica's parents would give the medication, but often they ended up in the hospital or doctor's office. They felt frustrated, scared, and alone. "We just didn't know what else to do. We couldn't understand why our little girl, who seemed otherwise so healthy and happy, could have such severe breathing problems." And all the while the doctors kept saying that Jessica would probably grow out of her condition.

When Jessica was almost five, her mother heard of a pediatrician in the area who specialized in asthma and allergies. Mary remembers being torn between thinking that this could be the answer they had been looking for and wondering whether the new doctor would tell her more of the same: that her daughter would eventually grow out of her condition. The pediatrician began by asking Mary about what medications Jessica was using. "I felt dumb," Mary says. "After all this time, all I knew was that we had a lot of different medications to use depending on what Jessica was feeling. I knew the names of some of them, but not all." With further questioning by the pediatrician, Mary also learned that she knew very little about what factors triggered Jessica's asthma attacks, about the possible side effects of Jessica's medications, or about what to do to prevent attacks or make them less severe.

After talking to Mary, the pediatrician performed a complete physical examination of Jessica, including tests of her lung function. When he was finished, he told Mary that Jessica had moderately severe asthma, that she would have this condition for the rest of her life, that there were drugs that she should take on a daily basis to lessen the severity and frequency of her attacks, that there was no reason Jessica should have to go to the hospital every time she had an asthma attack, and that there were many things Mary could do around the home to reduce Jessica's exposure to asthma triggers. "But the two most important things I remember are that he said that Jessica could lead a perfectly normal life even with her asthma, and my husband and I would become a team whose job it was to control Jessica's disease."

Mary had taken the first steps toward controlling her daughter's asthma. She learned that parents are an integral part of the asthma care program of their children. With that visit to a doctor trained in asthma, Mary learned that there were many things her family could do to help control Jessica's breathing. Perhaps the most important lesson was that Jessica was no different from other children and that with a properly designed asthma maintenance plan she could take part in almost any activity. "For the first time since Jessica's first asthma attack, I felt like we were in control," Mary says.

Jessica is now 13 and she is doing fine. She uses an inhaled steroid drug every day to reduce the underlying inflammation in her lungs and prevent many asthma attacks. She also has an inhaled beta-adrenergic drug to reverse occasional bouts of wheezing. Jessica and her family also know which asthma triggers she should avoid to reduce the chance that she has an asthma attack. Because of these measures, she plays sports with her friends, has an active social life, and is a perfectly normal young girl, but with asthma. "After all those years we were finally able to take control of her disease," Mary says. "And the biggest help was knowledge and understanding of the disease." ❑

erable coordination to use. A child must be able to press the canister of medication at the same time that he or she inhales the mist coming from the mouthpiece. Pressing the canister before inhaling may cause the asthma drug to be deposited in the child's mouth; pressing the canister after inhaling may cause the medication mist to go into the air rather than into the lungs. A number of devices have been developed that either eliminate the use of metered-dose inhalers for very young children under the ages of three or four or make these inhalers easier for children to use. All these devices have one purpose: getting adequate amounts of medication to the lungs of children with asthma.

Nebulizers

Compressor-driven nebulizers have been used to deliver asthma medications for years by hospital wards and emergency rooms. These machines are about the size of a bread box and consist of an air compressor attached to a tube. At the other end of the tube is a kind of holding canister for the medication with a mouthpiece. Nebulizers work by forcing air past the solution of medication in the holding canister and producing a fine mist. The child inhales this mist through a mouthpiece or face mask while breathing normally.

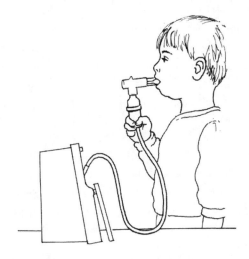

Nebulizers are a good alternative for young children who cannot master the intricacies of using a metered-dose inhaler.

Nebulizers can be a valuable tool in treating young children with asthma. Because the flow of medication through the mouthpiece or face mask is continual, children with asthma who cannot coordinate the use of a metered-dose inhaler can get adequate quantities of medications to their lungs. Home use of nebulizers has enabled parents to control their children's asthma without subjecting them to repeated trips to the hospital. Since children can be treated at home with drugs to reverse constriction of the airways or to prevent and reverse airway inflammation, their asthma attacks can be prevented or the severity of them lessened.

You should consider buying a nebulizer for use in your home after consulting with your doctor. Nebulizers may be useful for very young children with asthma and for children with poorly controlled or severe disease that requires frequent visits to the hospital. Many doctors recommend nebulizers only for very young children and only until the child becomes adept enough to use a metered-dose inhaler with a spacer, with or without a face mask.

Nebulizers have some drawbacks. They are cumbersome pieces of equipment that require electricity to run and therefore do not travel well. For this reason, doctors recommend that parents of children with asthma who are using a nebulizer also get an alternative form of treatment (such as a metered-dose inhaler with a spacer or dry powder inhaler) to use when away from home. There may also be a stigma attached to using nebulizers. Because these devices are large machines and children must sit and use them for 15 to 30 minutes at a time, some doctors feel that regularly using a nebulizer may impart a sense of dependence to children with asthma. Some children with asthma may feel that they are invalids who must always be in close proximity to their nebulizer. This sense of dependence is opposite to what children with asthma should be taught. They should be taught that asthma is a disease that needs to be controlled but that need not limit them from taking part in normal activities. That's why many doctors try to wean children off nebulizers as soon as possible, opting instead for metered-dose inhalers with spacers and face masks attached. Nonetheless, nebulizers are an important tool in managing childhood asthma. And they are one more way to take charge of your child's disease.

You can buy a nebulizer and the needed attachments, such as a face mask, for $180 to $260. Ask your doctor to recommend a brand of nebulizer, and shop around for the best price. Many medical device companies make nebulizers, and you can find them in most local medical supply stores and pharmacies. Many insurance plans will pay 80 percent of the cost.

Asthma medications—including adrenergic drugs to ease constriction of the airways, such as albuterol, and anti-inflammatory medications, such as cromolyn and nedocromil—are available in liquid form for use in a nebulizer. Parents may have to mix these drugs with a sterile saline solution to dilute them before using them in a nebulizer.

Face Masks

It often is difficult for children to coordinate the act of inhaling at precise times. This can be a problem when using a nebulizer or metered-dose inhaler. If your child does not breathe in when the medication is issuing forth from a nebulizer or metered-dose inhaler, the drug will not reach the lungs. Even when a child does coordinate inhalation with the delivery of the mist of medication, other problems can arise. To adequately disperse asthma medications in the lungs, doctors recommend that people with asthma hold their breath for a few seconds after inhaling. If your child does not do this, the medication may not have ample time to settle in the lungs and your child may require additional puffs of the drugs.

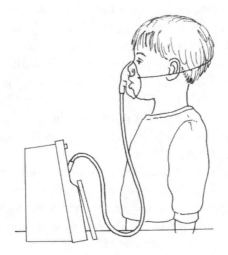

Face masks allow even very young children to benefit from inhaled asthma medicines.

Face masks can alleviate both of these problems. Face masks, attached to the mouthpieces on nebulizers and to spacer devices connected to metered-dose inhalers, are fastened to your child's face with an elastic band. When masks are used with a nebulizer, the flow of medication to the child's mouth is continual. Thus, with every breath your child takes, he or she is inhaling the asthma medication. When face masks are used with a metered-dose inhaler, they must be used in conjunction with a spacer. Spacers are discussed in more detail below.

A face mask, spacer, and metered-dose inhaler can allow the majority of children with asthma (even the very young) to avoid the use of a nebulizer. Parents fasten the face mask to the child's face and press the canister on the metered-dose inhaler. The medication mist is collected in the spacer, and when the child breathes, he or she inhales the medication. This also is a good way to train your child in using a metered-dose inhaler. The more your child sees how a metered-dose inhaler works, the more familiar he or she will be with the device. In time, as your child grows and can coordinate inhaling with pressing the canister on a metered-dose inhaler, you can do away with the face mask.

Spacers

We have seen that metered-dose inhalers can be tricky for a child to learn to coordinate. Even many adults with asthma do not use one properly. Spacers can help both children and adults with asthma get proper amounts of medication to their lungs by reducing the need for accurate coordination when using a metered-dose inhaler. Spacers are tubes that are attached to the mouthpiece of the inhaler. These tubes collect the mist of medication so that your child with asthma can inhale when he or she wants. Once in the spacer, the medication mist will not go anywhere, so your child does not have to breathe in at the exact time that he or she presses the metered-dose inhaler canister. Inhaling from a spacer allows your child to take in the asthma medication at a slower, more even rate.

Spacers are also used to reduce the possibility of side effects from asthma medications. The most common side effects associated with metered-dose inhalers are coughing, wheezing, dry mouth, and bad taste. Inhaled steroids also pose the risk of possible mouth infections. (For a detailed description of the side effects of asthma medications, see chapter 4.) All these side effects happen because much of the mist of asthma medication coming from a metered-dose inhaler can settle in the mouth unless the person using it precisely coordinates inhaling with pressing the canister of the inhaler. By collecting the medication mist before it is inhaled, spacers can help prevent many of these side effects. Studies have found that asthma medications inhaled through a spacer are more evenly distributed in the lungs, and less is collected in the mouth. And the air in the spacer dilutes the bad taste of some asthma medications.

There are many types of spacers available. Some are designed for specific asthma inhalers; others can be used with a wide range of metered-dose inhalers. There even is one inhaled steroid drug that comes in a metered-dose inhaler with its own spacer already built in. Ask your doctor about which spacer is best for your child. Two of the most popular spacers are the InspirEase and the Aerochamber.

InspirEase. The InspirEase spacer is a deflatable bag and mouthpiece into which you insert the end of your child's metered-dose inhaler.

When the canister on the metered-dose inhaler is depressed, the medication mist fills and inflates the InspirEase bag. This spacer has many advantages for young children who are taking their asthma medication under the supervision of their parents. If your child breathes the medication in too quickly, the bag will make a slight whistling sound. Since slow inhalation of asthma medication leads to better disbursement of the drug in the bronchioles, this is a helpful feedback feature for parents. And since the bag collapses as the child breathes in, the parent has a visual cue that the child is getting the medicine.

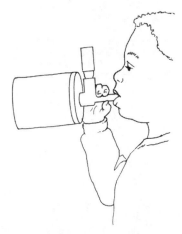

The collapsible InspirEase chamber helps children learn how to use a metered-dose inhaler, while allowing parents to monitor their breathing.

HOW TO USE AN INSPIREASE SPACER

1. Shake the canister.

2. Extend the bag.

3. Have the child place the mouthpiece of the metered-dose inhaler in his or her mouth and instruct the child to place the tongue over the mouthpiece.

4. Press the canister, allowing one puff of medication mist to enter the InspirEase chamber.

5. Have the child inhale slowly with lips around the mouthpiece and hold breath for up to 5 seconds.

6. Remove the mouthpiece and have your child breathe out slowly.

7. Wait about 2 minutes and repeat steps 1 through 5.

Aerochamber. The Aerochamber is a hard plastic tube with a mouth-piece or face mask on one end. The other end of the spacer is attached to your child's metered-dose inhaler. There is a one-way valve in the mouthpiece that prevents your child from exhaling back into the tube. For young children who cannot use a mouthpiece, the Aerochamber also comes with a face mask. When using the face mask, it is not possible for the parent to control the speed of inhalation or monitor whether the child actually is getting the medication.

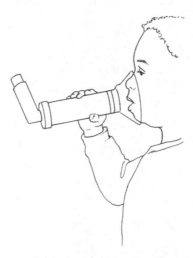

The Aerochamber inhaler is a solid tube that collects
the medication mist, making inhaling easier.

HOW TO USE THE AEROCHAMBER SPACER

1. Shake the canister.

2. Have the child place the mouthpiece of the Aerochamber in his or her mouth and close lips around it.

3. Press the canister of the metered-dose inhaler, allowing one puff of medication to enter the spacer.

4. Have your child inhale slowly and hold his or her breath for 5 seconds.

5. Tell your child to exhale slowly.

6. Wait about 2 minutes and repeat steps 1 through 4.

Dry Powder Inhalers

Some asthma medications are also available in so-called dry powder inhalers. These devices contain capsules or small pockets of powder asthma medication. With some devices, parents must open the inhaler and insert a new capsule for each inhalation. Others contain multiple capsules or pockets of medication. With multiple-use inhalers, parents simply turn the base of the inhaler until a click is heard, signifying that the mouthpiece has been moved over to the next dose of asthma medication.

DID YOU KNOW...?

Metered-dose inhalers for asthma are going green. The reason for the eco-switch is the chlorofluorocarbons, or CFCs, used to propel asthma medications from the canisters of metered-dose inhalers. Some environmental scientists believe these chemicals are helping to deplete the earth's ozone layer. Global warming is blamed on depletion of the ozone layer.

Many of the world's nations, including the United States, have agreed to stop using CFCs, with the exception of products considered essential. Asthma inhalers are one such product that has been granted a temporary exemption to the ban on CFCs. In the meantime, drug companies are looking for other ways to deliver asthma medications. The problem is to come up with another type of propellant that can make a mist of asthma medications fine enough to travel deep into the lungs when inhaled. The first aerosol inhaler that does not contain CFCs was approved by the U.S. Food and Drug Administration in 1996.

Drug companies are investigating everything from new propellants to metered-dose inhalers that use no propellants to new types of dry powder inhalers. The ideal dry powder inhaler of the future would hold many doses of medication, just as the current crop of metered-dose inhalers holds many inhalations of asthma medication.

It is unclear what the future of metered-dose inhalers will be, but one thing is for sure: in the future, no one will be able to say that your asthma inhaler is hurting the ozone layer.

Dry powder inhalers have some advantages over metered-dose inhalers, especially for use by children. There is no need to coordinate releasing the medication and breathing when using a dry powder inhaler; these devices are activated by your child's breath—that is, the medication is released by the force of your child inhaling on the mouthpiece. All the child has to do is inhale, and medication surges through the mouthpiece into his or her lungs. But dry powder inhalers do have some disadvantages. Unlike metered-dose inhalers that deliver a fine mist of medication, these devices use a dry powder form of the medication. Some of this powder may become deposited in the mouth, and some children complain about the taste. There is also some concern about how well dry powder inhalers actually get medication to the lungs. Doctors are still studying the devices to determine if the needed amount of the powder reaches the bronchioles, where it can relieve constriction and inflammation.

Asthma Drugs for Children

As we have seen, many of the asthma drugs used by adults are also used by children, but in different forms so that they can be inhaled through a nebulizer or dry powder inhaler or taken orally in pill or liquid form. (A detailed description of asthma drugs and their possible side effects is given in chapter 4.) Let's look at some of the differences in the commonly used children's asthma medications.

Adrenergic drugs for children are available in pill or liquid form to be taken orally; in metered-dose inhalers, which can be used with spacers and face masks; and in liquid form for use in a nebulizer. The adrenergic drugs most commonly used for children are albuterol, metaproterenol, terbutaline, bitolterol, and pirbuteral.

Steroids are available for children with asthma in either a pill (for oral use) or in metered-dose inhalers (which can be used with spacers and face masks). Unfortunately, there are no liquid steroids available in the United States for use in a nebulizer for children. This means that the parents of children who need an inhaled steroid to reduce their lung inflammation must take an active part in their treatment.

Most children—even very young children under the age of four—can use a steroid metered-dose inhaler with a spacer and face mask. But young children who need inhaled steroids need extra help until they become adept at coordinating the use of a metered-dose inhaler. Parents can provide this help by becoming partners in their child's asthma treatment. You can start by helping your child use a steroid metered-dose inhaler with a spacer and face mask. Attach the face mask, press the canister, and monitor how he or she inhales the asthma drug. As your child grows, you may be able to do away with the face mask, and eventually he or she will be able to use an inhaler alone.

Most children can use a steroid metered-dose inhaler with a spacer, face mask, and parental help. If this approach is not working with your child, talk to your doctor. Although they are not approved by the Food and Drug Administration for this use, some doctors advise parents to use liquid steroids contained in nose sprays for use in a nebulizer and they can instruct parents in how this is done. While this is effective for some children with asthma, doctors do not know for sure if the steroids contained in nose sprays are completely safe when used in a nebulizer. You should talk to your doctor about this possibility if your child requires inhaled steroids and cannot master using a metered-dose inhaler.

The jury still is out on whether inhaled steroids retard growth rates in children. Studies of children with asthma taking inhaled steroids are evenly divided between those showing that inhaled steroids have no effect on growth rates and those finding that the drugs can suppress growth. What is known is that for children with severe asthma, the undesirable effects of not using an inhaled steroid to reduce airway inflammation and reduce the chance of severe asthma attacks far outweigh any possible effects on the child's growth rate.

Cromolyn and nedocromil are used frequently to treat children with asthma. These drugs come in metered-dose inhalers and a liquid form for use in a nebulizer. Doctors will often try one of these drugs on a child with asthma before resorting to an inhaled steroid because both drugs have minimal side effects and are very safe. Cromolyn and nedocromil can reduce airway inflammation in children with asthma and may prevent some attacks of wheezing brought on by exercise or exposure to allergens.

Theophylline is an oral drug that is available in pill form or liquid for use in children. It can relieve constriction in the airways, allowing them to open more widely and ease breathing, and may reduce and prevent nighttime attacks of wheezing. Theophylline can cause children to be excited, restless, and agitated. Some studies have even suggested that theophylline may also cause learning problems in children, but the new thinking is that any learning problems associated with theophylline are probably the result of the drug's other side effects. That is, if the drug causes a child to be restless and excited, that child will probably have trouble sitting still in class. Many children who require this drug can avoid those problems by taking a slow-release version of the drug, which enters the bloodstream slowly and evenly, or by taking the medication late in the afternoon or early evening.

Your doctor will want to periodically check the level of theophylline in your child's blood.

A Step-by-Step Approach to Treating Asthma in Children Over 5

The same classifications of the severity of asthma in adults also apply to asthma in children over 5. New guidelines published by the federal government's National Asthma Education and Prevention Program in 1997 classify asthma in four degrees of severity: mild intermittent, mild persistent, moderate persistent, and severe persistent. The guidelines include a suggested step-by-step approach to treating the different classes of asthma severity.

Mild Intermittent Asthma

Characterized by symptoms two or fewer times a week, two or fewer episodes of nighttime asthma symptoms per month, and lung function at 80 percent of normal or greater. Asthma flare-ups are brief (from a few hours to a few days); intensity may vary.

Daily Medication: No daily medication is needed

Quick Relief: Inhaled beta$_2$-agonists as needed for symptoms.

Mild Persistent Asthma

Characterized by symptoms more than twice a week but less than once every day; nighttime symptoms more than twice a month, and lung function at 80 percent of normal or greater. Asthma flare-ups may affect activity.

Daily Medication: Either low doses of inhaled corticosteroid, or cromolyn or nedocromil. Children usually begin with a trial of cromolyn or nedocromil. Sustained-release theophylline is an alternative. Zafirlukast or zileuton may also be considered for patients 12 years of age or older.

Quick Relief: Inhaled beta$_2$-agonists as needed for symptoms.

Moderate Persistent Asthma

Characterized by daily symptoms and daily use of inhaled short-acting beta$_2$-agonists; nighttime symptoms more than once a week, and lung function at 60 percent to 80 percent of normal. Asthma flare-ups affect activity; they occur two or more times a week and may last days.

Daily Medication: Either inhaled corticosteroid (medium dose) or inhaled corticosteroid (low–medium dose) and a long-acting bronchodilator, especially for nighttime symptoms: either long-acting beta$_2$-agonists, sustained-release theophylline, or long-acting beta$_2$-agonist tablets. If needed: anti-inflammatory inhaled corticosteroids (medium–high dose) AND long-acting bronchodilator, especially for nighttime symptoms: either long-acting inhaled beta$_2$-agonists, sustained-release theophylline, or long-acting beta$_2$-agonist tablets.

Quick Relief: Inhaled beta$_2$-agonists as needed for symptoms.

Severe Persistent Asthma

Characterized by continual symptoms, limited physical activity, and frequent asthma flare-ups; frequent nighttime symptoms; and lung function at 60 percent of normal or less.

Daily Medication: Inhaled corticosteroid (high dose) and either long-acting inhaled beta$_2$-agonists, sustained-release theophylline, or long-acting beta$_2$-agonist tablets AND corticosteroid tablets or syrup long term.

Quick Relief: Inhaled beta$_2$-agonists as needed for symptoms.

For infants and young childen, the NAEPP guidelines suggest that doctors may try inhaled bronchodilators and anti-inflammatory medications. When initiating daily anti-inflammatory therapy for babies or young children, cromolyn or nedocromil is often tried.

An Asthma Emergency Plan

An asthma emergency plan for children is as important as one for adults. You should know ahead of time what to do during different phases when your child is having an asthma attack. When you see your child having breathing problems, you may not be able to think clearly and may feel overly rushed to come up with a solution. By having a well-documented plan that you can refer to during different phases of an asthma attack, you will know precisely what steps to take. You should talk to your child's doctor about developing such a plan, which might be based on your child's peak flow readings. You can use the asthma management plan in chapter 4 when you discuss devising one for your child. Make sure you ask the doctor about what steps to take if your child's peak flow measurements enter the red zone. This is a danger area, and you should have a predetermined course of action to take.

6 / Trigger-Proofing Your Life

ASTHMA IS A DISEASE THAT MUST BE CONTROLLED. WE ALREADY have learned that monitoring asthma, by becoming familiar with the signs of an impending asthma attack and by observing lung function with peak flow testing, can lead to better awareness of when an attack may strike. Once armed with that knowledge, you are better able to judge when to use asthma medications to cut short, or even prevent, attacks of wheezing. People with moderate to severe asthma must also control their disease by regularly taking asthma medications that reduce the underlying inflammation in their lungs. As we have learned, these medications must be taken even when you are not having trouble breathing. After reading this book, talking with your doctor, and following some simple steps outlined in these pages, you can reduce the chances that you will suffer repeated asthma attacks.

While monitoring asthma symptoms and controlling breathing with medications are effective (and indeed essential) for most people with asthma, they are only part of a total asthma care program. Another fundamental aspect to controlling asthma is avoiding or reducing exposure to the promoters and triggers that can cause airway inflammation, constriction, and ultimately, wheezing. As we have seen, asthma promoters and triggers are essential in the process that leads to an asthma attack. Without these promoters and triggers, no person with asthma would experience bouts of breathing difficulties. Consequently, an integral part of any asthma care program is reducing or eliminating your exposure to these promoters and triggers.

This part of an asthma care program is often referred to as environmental control. Doctors now believe that many people with asthma can significantly reduce the number of attacks they will have by implementing environmental control over asthma triggers in their homes, in their schools, and while traveling. In this chapter you will learn of steps you can take to reduce the number of asthma triggers in and around your home. By following the advice in this chapter, you can significantly reduce the chance that you will encounter asthma triggers while at home. (Environmental controls in schools and while traveling are discussed further in chapters 14 and 16.)

Many of these steps are simple. Yet their effect can be great. Environmental control of asthma promoters and triggers is the best prevention available for derailing asthma attacks before they start. It also is the form of asthma care that is the safest; the only side effect to regularly washing sheets in hot water, for instance, is probably inconvenience. While the most carefully adhered to environmental control plan cannot rid your home of asthma promoters and triggers completely, following these measures can take you one step closer to trigger-proofing your home and your life.

Asthma Promoters and Triggers

Asthma promoters and triggers are either irritants that cause constriction of the airways or allergens that cause the body's immune system to mount an attack ultimately leading to inflammation of the airways. However they work, you should strive as much as possible to rid your home and life of these promoters and triggers. In addition to triggering an asthma attack, allergens can also cause the misery of watery eyes and runny nose with which people with allergic rhinitis are all too familiar. Other options, such as immunotherapy injections and antihistamine drugs, also should be employed to reduce the effect of allergens. (More information on how to control allergies is given in chapters 8 and 9.)

There recently has been a heightened awareness of the importance of controlling asthma promoters and triggers in the home. This is linked to the growing observation that recently constructed houses can act to trap asthma promoters and triggers. Wall-to-wall carpeting, insulation to reduce heat loss, and decreased ventilation from tight-fitting windows and doors all act to trap asthma promoters and triggers inside. Recognizing these shifts in the ways we live, many asthma specialists have begun to recommend that the families of people with asthma aggressively pursue ways to reduce the levels of promoters and triggers in their homes. We'll review some of the common asthma promoters and triggers in the home and suggest steps you can take to virtually trigger-proof your home.

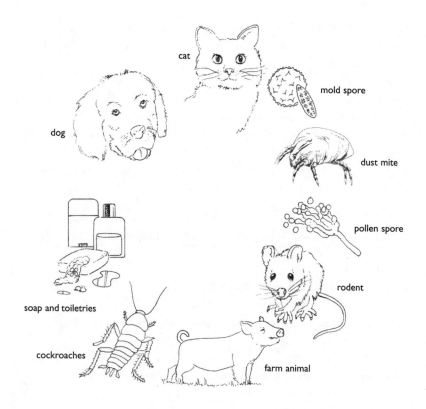

*Furry animals, cockroaches, dust mites, pollen, viruses,
and scented deodorants all can trigger an asthma attack.*

Dust Mites

Dust mites are one of the most important asthma triggers. For years doctors and patients have known that some people with asthma can have an attack triggered by exposure to dust. This commonly was called a house dust allergy. But researchers have found that people are not allergic to the dust itself. Tiny insects, called house dust mites, are now known to trigger these asthma attacks.

Mites live in specks of dust. As we have seen in chapter 3, mites can trigger an asthma attack by causing IgE antibodies to react, latch onto mast cells, and cause these cells to release irritating and inflammatory substances. The resulting explosion releases chemicals that cause the airways to become inflamed. Dust mites look like microscopic versions of ticks and spiders. They grow best where it is warm and humid and live on a diet of human skin particles found throughout your house.

Dust mites can live in surface dust, but their preferred home is fabric (that on mattresses, pillows, bedding, carpets, upholstered furniture, and stuffed animals).

There are three ways you can try to lower the number of dust mites sharing your home: (1) remove objects in which they live, such as carpets, upholstered furniture, and stuffed animals; (2) wrap some of these objects (such as mattresses and pillows) in protective covers so the mites cannot get out; and (3) try to wash them out of some objects, such as bed sheets. An aggressive environmental control program aimed at dust mites uses all three approaches.

TIPS FOR CONTROLLING DUST MITES

Things to do first
➤ Cover mattresses and pillows.
➤ Remove stuffed animals from the bedroom.
➤ Remove upholstered furniture and fabric-covered items from the bedroom.
➤ Wet-mop floors.
➤ Vacuum regularly, using special allergen-controlling bags or machines.
➤ Improve ventilation.
➤ Stop using humidifiers.
➤ Place filters over heating vents.

Things to do next
➤ Remove carpets, especially in the bedrooms and basement.
➤ Dehumidify.

Things to do last
➤ Use air cleaners.
➤ Use air filters on heating ducts.
➤ Use chemicals that kill mites and destroy allergens.

You should begin controlling dust mites in the bedroom, where mites thrive in mattresses and bedding. Encase mattresses and pillows in airtight plastic or vinyl covers, which can be purchased at most department stores and through mail order companies. A cover adequate to control dust mites should encase the entire mattress or pillow and should zipper shut. Special allergy-proof cases are made out of a special soft material or with a layer of fabric that is more comfortable to sleep on than crinkly plastic or vinyl. You can also try putting a mattress pad on top of these covers to make them more comfortable. Mattress and pillow covers should be cleaned once a week with a damp cloth or sponge.

The next step to controlling dust mites is to consider removing all unnecessary fabric items from the bedroom. Try to get rid of as many stuffed animals as possible. You should also remove extra pillows, canopies, and thick comforters (especially down comforters) and replace them with items you can readily wash. You should wash all bedding in hot water at least once every two weeks to kill mites. Most scientists agree that washing at a temperature of 130°F can kill up to 90 percent of mites.

The next issue in dust mite control is carpets. It is probably a good idea to get rid of any area carpets except for those that you can easily wash. When it comes to wall-to-wall carpeting, the decision is more difficult. This can be an expensive procedure, especially in newer homes that do not have usable flooring under the carpeting. There is also a safety consideration. If you have young children in your family, you will have to weigh the danger of hard flooring against the need to reduce mite contamination. Very young children can get injured by falling on hard flooring, and wall-to-wall carpeting reduces this risk. Therefore you should probably resort to removing your wall-to-wall carpeting only after you or your family member with asthma has been found to be allergic to dust mites and you have tried other measures to reduce the levels of mites in your home.

Frequent vacuuming and shampooing are suggested as alternatives to removing wall-to-wall carpeting. While vacuuming can reduce mite levels in carpets, it still cannot get at them all. Nonetheless, vacuuming is a good alternative to taking up your carpeting. The downside to vacuuming is that most vacuums blow particles throughout the air and can actually kick up asthma promoters and triggers that linger for 1 to 2 hours after vacuuming. There are two solutions to this problem. Many companies now sell special allergy bags that fit in most commercial vacuum cleaners. These bags have much smaller openings than traditional vacuum bags, thus reducing the amount of particles blown into the air. Another option is to buy a vacuum cleaner with a special HEPA (High Efficiency Particulate Air) filter that traps particles before they are blown back into the air.

One reason for increased concentrations of household mites is the trend toward tighter, more energy-efficient homes that have less ventilation. You can counter the effects of this by adequately ventilating your house, even by just opening the windows periodically. You also should strive to keep your house as dry as possible. The tiny mite grows best when the relative humidity is above 55 percent. Although the relative humidity of your home depends in large part on the area of the country in which you live, you can control humidity by limiting the use of humidifiers and by using air conditioning, which dries out the air.

If after taking these steps you are still bothered by dust mites in the home, you may want to resort to three additional environmental control measures: (1) have the heating and air-conditioning ducts in your home fitted with air filters; (2) buy a stand-alone HEPA air filter that draws air in and filters out particles; and (3) clean your carpets and upholstered furniture with products that kill mites. One such product, benzyl benzoate, is sold in a moist powder that can be sprinkled on furniture and carpets and then vacuumed up.

When trying to control the amount of dust mites in your home, consult the table on page 78. You should begin by following the table in order. You may find that mites are adequately controlled before completing all the steps listed.

"Anthony"

By the time their second son, Anthony, was born, his parents knew about as much about asthma and allergies as they could hope to know. Anthony was born a little more than three years after Joe, so their parents, John and Angie, already had about two and a half years of investigation under their belts. They already knew that asthma and allergies ran in the family, and they already had the experience of going from doctor to doctor before Joe's breathing problems were properly diagnosed.

So they were prepared for the possibility that their second son would follow in the footsteps of their first, down the road of asthma and allergies. And indeed that's just what happened. Anthony's first asthma attack happened when he was about one year old. As he was lying in the crib one day, Angie heard a telltale wheeze emanating from his tiny lungs. "I knew what it was right away because we had already been through this," she recalls.

The house was already devoid of most asthma triggers because of their experience with Joe. There were few stuffed toys in the bedrooms, and the family never kept any pets. Carpeting was at a minimum, and the house was kept as dust free as possible. But it seemed that the influence of the family's genes was too strong to overcome.

Anthony was taken to the pediatrician after that first asthma attack and was promptly placed on regular doses of theophylline to control his airways. His mother, Angie, was certain that armed with the knowledge she had gained from Joe's bout with asthma, she would be prepared for anything Anthony could throw at her. But what she found was that asthma and allergies affect everyone differently, even members of the same family.

Whereas Joe seemed to wheeze more during exercise or activities, Anthony had more trouble at night. While Joe was horrendously bothered by hay fever in the spring and ragweed pollen in the fall, Anthony, though he did suffer many of the same symptoms, such as itching and a runny nose, seemed less troubled. And while certain foods caused Joe to break out in hives and occasionally wheeze, Anthony could eat anything put in front of him, and he often did.

Growing up, Joe and Anthony took care of each other. In school, recess meant that the brothers would keep an eye out for each other to see if there were any signs of exercise-induced asthma.

While both brothers had the same disease, the triggers that caused them to have breathing problems were quite different. "I thought I was going to know what to expect, but it turns out that all my boys are different, from their personalities to what causes their asthma to flare up," Angie says. Since asthma is a disease of triggers, recognizing these triggers and taking steps to reduce exposure to them is of primary importance. What the family learned is that just because one family member with asthma or allergies responds to certain triggers, that doesn't mean other affected family members will react in the same way or at all. "In the beginning it's a little confusing, but in a family you learn to live with it, and as your children grow older, they recognize their own disease," Angie says. "The biggest thing is to teach your children about their disease, what they need to do to control it, and how they can treat it if they have an asthma attack."

So individualized is this disease that when John and Angie's third son, Val, was born a little more than a year after Anthony, the family soon discovered that he has perhaps the worst allergic rhinitis of any of the brothers but to date has no signs of asthma. Nevertheless, there are some triggers that affect all the brothers. Anthony and Joe both wheeze when they get a cold or flu; none can stand to be around animals like cats and dogs or they start sneezing, itching, and having runny noses and teary eyes (Anthony and Joe also begin to wheeze and cough); and being around a smoker causes symptoms in all three. ❑

Animal Allergens

Furry animals such as cats and dogs; rodents, including rats, rabbits, and guinea pigs; and farm animals such as horses and cows can all cause allergies and trigger an asthma attack. It is estimated that between 5 and 10 percent of people in the United States are allergic to one or more animals. Animal allergens can promote asthma attacks by leading to lung inflammation, can trigger attacks in people with already inflamed lungs, and can cause allergy symptoms such as allergic rhinitis and watery eyes. Unfortunately, there are no safe breeds of animals for people with asthma or allergies. Even so-called short-hair and non-shedding breeds of cats and dogs can cause allergies and trigger asthma attacks. The most common animal allergens are saliva, urine, and secretions from glands in the animal's skin. These substances become airborne when the animal sheds, and even the shortest-hair breeds do shed.

If you or someone in your family has asthma or allergies to animals, you probably should not have a pet. But this is an emotional decision that is often based on many factors besides the effects of having an animal in your home. Pets become part of the family and are often difficult to give up. If you or someone in your family has asthma or allergies and you are unwilling to give up your pet, there are some things you can do to reduce the levels of animal allergens in your home. None of these environmental controls will rid your home of animal allergens, but they can reduce their levels. If after trying them you find that you or your family member with asthma or allergies still is suffering repeated attacks, you may have to rethink your decision to keep your pets.

TIPS FOR CONTROLLING ANIMAL ALLERGIES

➤ Keep pets outdoors as much as possible.
➤ When indoors, keep pets in the kitchen or other uncarpeted areas.
➤ Keep pets out of the bedroom.
➤ Remove carpeting and upholstered furniture, especially in the bedroom.
➤ Keep bedroom doors closed.
➤ Provide good ventilation.
➤ Use an air cleaner.
➤ Wash your pet regularly.
➤ If you are allergic, have someone else brush and groom the pet.

Many of the steps recommended to control the levels of dust mites will also help to reduce the levels of animal allergens in your home.

These include regular vacuuming, ventilating your home, getting rid of upholstered furniture and carpeting, especially in the bedroom, and using HEPA air filters to clean the air of animal allergens. One study by researchers in the United Kingdom found that levels of dog allergens were reduced in rooms with HEPA air filters compared to rooms that did not have the filters. But people with asthma or allergies who keep pets should also try other environmental control measures.

You should keep pets outdoors as much as possible. This will reduce the amount of animal hair contaminated with saliva, urine, and other secretions that can become airborne in your home. If you do bring your pet indoors, you should keep it out of the bedroom and in areas of the home that do not have carpeting or upholstered furniture. When your pet is indoors, you should make sure that the bedroom doors are closed. You should also limit the activities between your family member with asthma or allergies and your pet. Have another family member wash and groom the pet.

Regularly washing a pet may reduce the levels of allergens in its fur. One study by researchers in the United Kingdom found that washing dogs with shampoo under a shower reduced by sixfold the levels of allergens in the dogs' fur. Researchers do not know how often you must wash your pet or how effective a sixfold reduction in allergens is in preventing asthma attacks and allergy symptoms. If you do decide to give up your pet, you should wash your home thoroughly after the animal leaves. Animal allergens are notoriously difficult to get rid of; it may take several cleanings to rid your home of leftover animal allergens.

Cockroaches

We have seen that cockroaches are very potent asthma triggers. This is especially true in homes in the inner city. Sensitivity to cockroach allergens is an especially important asthma trigger in children. The National Cooperative Inner City Asthma Study examined the homes of 611 children with asthma between the ages of four and nine who lived in large metropolitan areas. The study found high levels of cockroach allergens in 89 percent of the children's bedrooms.

Environmental control of cockroach allergens is notoriously difficult. The first step is aggressive extermination. You can try to do this yourself with a number of commercially available products, or you can hire an exterminator. Roach traps, pesticide bombs, and spray insecticides can all be tried in areas of typical cockroach pathways, for example, around kitchen cabinets and drawers. Boric acid powder is highly effective in killing cockroaches and can be spread under stoves, refrigerators, and other areas where roaches hide.

TIPS FOR CONTROLLING COCKROACHES

➤ Aggressively exterminate your home.

➤ Thoroughly clean your home after extermination.

➤ Seal entry points to prevent reinfestation.

➤ Do not store grocery bags, cardboard boxes, newspapers, or empty bottles in your home.

After exterminating, the next step is to clean your home thoroughly to rid it of dead roaches. As we learned in chapter 3, when dead roaches decompose, their body parts become aerosolized. These tiny flakes can become inhaled and trigger an asthma attack. After cleaning your home, you should try to prevent roaches from returning by sealing all entry points. You should repair cracks and holes in walls, floors, and window and door screens, and apply caulking around pipes that might provide a way in for roaches. Make sure you keep food in closed containers and wash all dishes and utensils immediately. It is important to repair leaky faucets, since cockroaches are attracted to moisture, and do not store grocery bags, cardboard boxes, newspapers, or empty bottles in your home, since these are the favored haunts of cockroaches.

Molds

Molds are microscopic fungi that can grow both indoors and out-doors. Indoors, molds are responsible for the unsightly mildew on bathroom tiles. Indoor molds are also found in basements, attics, refrigerators, garbage containers, carpets, and upholstery. Outdoors, molds grow on leaves, trees, and rotting wood. The spores of molds—in effect, baby molds—float in the air like pollen. Outdoor mold spores begin to grow after the spring thaw and reach their peak in July, August, September, and October in the northern United States. Outside molds can be found year-round in the South and along the West Coast.

You can control indoor molds by locating and eliminating as many breeding grounds as possible, keeping humidity levels in your home low, and killing molds where they are growing. As with dust mites, molds grow best in moist areas. You should begin by getting rid of carpeting and upholstered furniture in the basement, where humidity levels are higher. You should also get rid of any rug or fabric that has a musty smell or has had water damage. Go easy on the number of indoor house plants you have, since molds can grow in the soil.

TIPS FOR CONTROLLING MOLDS

➤ Identify areas of mold growth and clean them with fungicides or diluted chlorine bleach.

➤ Get rid of carpets and upholstered furniture in the basement.

➤ Limit use of humidifiers and use a dehumidifier, especially in the basement.

➤ Limit outdoor activities on days when mold levels are high.

➤ Don't rake leaves or garden in areas where there is significant mold growth.

Next, you should try to keep the relative humidity of your home below 50 percent to discourage mold growth. You can accomplish this by limiting the use of humidifiers and using a dehumidifier if you live in areas that are often humid or wet. Air conditioners are a good way to keep homes dry, but you should regularly wash the filters because they can become contaminated with molds.

The most common areas in your home where molds will grow are the basement walls and floors, window moldings, shower curtains, and bathroom walls and fixtures. Molds in these areas are usually easy to spot, as they may appear as a black, brown, or reddish substance. Once you have located molds in your home, clean the area with a fungicide cleaning product that kills molds on contact. You can also clean with a mixture of one part of chlorine bleach to 10 parts of water. An effective way of getting rid of molds on your shower curtain is to wash the curtain with some towels in the hot cycle with a cup of bleach. (Do not put a vinyl shower curtain in the dryer.)

You can't rid the outdoors of molds, but you can reduce your exposure to them. If you or your family member with asthma is sensitive to molds, you should limit outdoor activities when mold levels are high. Your local newspaper probably lists levels of mold along with pollution levels. Airborne levels of mold spores reach their peak on dry, windy days when the air kicks up mold spores that have been growing in moist areas. Raking leaves is not advised for people with asthma who have mold allergies; molds grow on downed leaves, and raking can stir up the spores.

Pollen

Pollen consists of tiny microscopic granules from trees, grasses, and weeds that are necessary for plant fertilization. When airborne, pollen can trigger asthma attacks and cause the symptoms of allergic rhinitis. (Allergic rhinitis is discussed further in chapter 8.) Different plants pollinate at different times of the year. The pollen of trees such as oak, western red cedar, elm, birch, ash, hickory, poplar, sycamore, maple, cypress, and walnut are often the cause of asthma attacks and allergic rhinitis symptoms in the early spring. During the late spring and early summer, pollinating grasses such as timothy, Bermuda, orchard, sweet vernal, red top, and bluegrass often are the culprits. As we move into the late summer and early fall, weed pollen tends to take over. The most common weed pollens that can trigger an asthma attack and cause allergic rhinitis symptoms are ragweed, sagebrush, pigweed, tumbleweed, Russian thistle, and cockleweed.

Every plant pollinates at a different period of the year. The pollination season starts earlier in the South, beginning as early as January, and starts later in the spring as you move north. In general, the pollen season lasts from February or March through October. Various groups and government agencies publish pollen counts each day during the pollen season. These counts measure how many grains of pollen there are per cubic meter of air. Many people with asthma or allergies can develop pollen-related symptoms when pollen counts are between 20 and 100 grains per cubic meter of air. However, even lower pollen counts can work to trigger an asthma attack by making sufferers more prone to the effects of other allergens.

TIPS FOR CONTROLLING EXPOSURE TO POLLEN

➤ Ventilate homes when pollen levels are low or after 10 A.M.

➤ Use air conditioners during pollen season.

➤ Limit outdoor activities when pollen levels are high.

➤ Wear a particle mask when doing yard work.

There is no way you can completely avoid pollen. But you can take some steps to reduce exposure. The first step requires a compromise in how you control the levels of dust mites and animal allergens in your home, that is, by carefully deciding when you will ventilate your home. We have seen that adequate ventilation can reduce the levels of dust mites and animal allergens, but if you decide to ventilate your home when pollen levels are high, you could be trading one allergen for another. A good compromise is to try not to ventilate your home when pollen levels are high—that is, when pollen counts are between 20 and 100 grains per cubic meter of air. You should also try ventilating your home after 10 A.M. because pollen levels are highest between 5 and 10 A.M. Using air conditioners during the pollen season is also a good compromise. Air conditioners keep the air in your home dry, thus reducing the levels of dust mites and molds, and they filter the outside air of pollen.

You should also limit outdoor activities when pollen levels are high. This is especially true for strenuous activities, such as hiking or exercise. When you exercise, you breathe more often and more deeply. If pollen counts are high, you will increase the amount of pollen inhaled. This is not to say that you should stay indoors throughout the entire pollen season. Stretch out your time indoors to minimize the amount of time spent outdoors. You should also try avoiding outdoor activities before 10 A.M., when pollen counts are at their highest. Also, try to avoid exercising in meadows, where irritating grasses and weeds grow, and shower and wash your hair afterward. Washing the pollen off, especially from your hair, is important, since it can rub off on your pillow and trigger asthma and allergies overnight. You also should take two puffs of inhaled cromolyn or nedocromil before exercising to reduce the effects of inhaled pollens, or your doctor may suggest using your beta-adrenergic inhaler before exercise. Antihistamines taken before outdoor activities also tend to reduce pollen-related asthma attacks and allergies. (More information about antihistamines is given in chapter 9.)

Indoor Irritants

Most of the agents discussed so far trigger an asthma attack or allergy symptoms because they are allergens. But there are numerous substances in the home that can trigger an asthma attack by irritating the airways and causing them to constrict. These substances are not allergens and thus do not cause allergy symptoms, but they still are asthma triggers that you can control by implementing some environmental control measures.

The most common indoor irritants that trigger asthma are passive smoke, nitrogen dioxide, wood smoke, and heavy cooking odors and smoke. You or your family member with asthma may also be bothered by heavily scented soaps, perfumes, or deodorants. We'll review these indoor irritants and what you can do to lower their levels and reduce the chance that they will trigger an attack.

There is little doubt that passive tobacco smoke is the most dangerous indoor irritant for people with asthma. A study published by the American Lung Association found that children between the ages of two and four who live in homes where one family member smokes are 280 percent more likely to wheeze than children from non-smoking families. After age five, the risk of persistent wheezing is still at an alarming 180 percent higher than among children from non-smoking homes. Besides increasing the risk of asthma, passive tobacco smoke has been linked to increases in the number and severity of virtually all respiratory disorders, including allergic rhinitis, bronchitis, pneumonia, and infections of the ear, upper respiratory tract, and nose.

The one environmental control for passive smoke is don't smoke. The evidence that tobacco smoke is hazardous to your health is overwhelming. When people with asthma are concerned, these effects are magnified. If you or your family member has asthma and someone in your household smokes, you should encourage the smoker to quit. If quitting is not an option, you should ban smoking in your home. Smoke-free homes are the best environmental control for passive smoke.

Nitrogen dioxide is a gas that is released from gas ranges, pilot lights, and many kerosene and gas heaters. About 50 percent of homes in the United States use gas for cooking appliances, so exposure to nitrogen dioxide is quite common. Exposure to high levels of nitrogen dioxide can decrease lung function and trigger coughing and wheezing. The first step in reducing levels of nitrogen dioxide is to avoid the use of kerosene space heaters. If you cook with gas and someone in your family has asthma, you should try to ventilate the kitchen as much as possible.

Smoke created from wood-burning ovens or stoves can be a significant asthma trigger. Wood smoke releases a variety of particles into the air, as well as carbon monoxide and other gases. If you have a wood-burning stove, check it for leaks. While some efficient models leak very little smoke into the home, other older or less efficient models can be more hazardous to your health. Fortunately, leaking stoves can be sealed around the edges and where the stove attaches to the chimney, thus reducing the levels of wood smoke pollutants in your home.

Some people with asthma may also be bothered by heavy cooking odors or smoke, scented soaps and perfumes, or some deodorants. The key issue here is avoidance. If you or your family member with asthma is bothered by certain scents, try using unscented soaps and antiperspirants. Heavy cooking odors or smoke should be ventilated from the kitchen as thoroughly as possible.

7 / The Link Between Asthma and Allergies

ASTHMA AND ALLERGIES ARE ONE OF THE GREAT PAIRS OF ALL TIME. Like Fred Astaire and Ginger Rogers, Antony and Cleopatra, or hot dogs and a baseball game, asthma and allergies are virtually inseparable. This companionship holds true for many aspects of these maladies, from how they affect the body to how they are treated. As doctors have uncovered some of the mysteries surrounding asthma and allergies, they have become more convinced of the intricate interplay between them, an interplay that holds important considerations for people with asthma or allergies.

The relationship between asthma and allergies runs deep. Both affect the airways. The airways are divided into two interrelated parts, the upper airway and the lower airway. In reality, however, the airway is one continuous path beginning with the mouth and nose and ending with the lungs. We have already seen how asthma affects the lower airway. In this chapter we will explore the relationship between the two airways and how allergies that affect the upper airway can trigger an asthma attack in the lower airway.

But the asthma-allergy link does not stop there. As we have seen, many asthma promoters and triggers work their harm in people with asthma by stimulating IgE antibodies. This increased production of IgE causes mast cells to release a variety of inflammatory chemicals that cause the airways to constrict and become swollen. The IgE response is the allergic response; that is, the system responds when provoked by allergens. In this chapter we'll also take a closer look at the IgE system and how it controls allergies and asthma.

More than 80 percent of people with asthma are allergic to one or more allergens. These allergy-causing substances can be pollen, molds, animal dander, dust mites, cockroaches, foods, medications, or stinging insect bites. The most common allergy is a condition known as allergic rhinitis, more commonly called hay fever. While not everyone with asthma also has hay fever, in those plagued by both conditions, hay fever can be a potent asthma trigger. Stimulated mast cells in the upper airway lead to the misery of runny nose and watery eyes; in the lower airway these mast cells and the chemicals they release can trigger an asthma attack and the wheezing and coughing that accompany these attacks. (More information about allergic rhinitis appears in chapter 8.) Molds, animal dander, dust mites, and cockroaches can work in the same way, triggering hay fever–like symptoms in the upper airway and asthma attacks in the lower airway.

Allergens do not have to affect the airways to trigger an asthma attack. Some substances such as foods, medications, and stinging insect bites work systemically—that is, the allergen can be in the digestive tract (in the case of foods and medications) or in the skin (via stinging insect bites). These types of allergic reactions may cause people with allergies to break out in hives. While these types of allergic reactions generally do not cause an asthma attack, they can lead to swelling throughout the body. This swelling can also affect the lower airway, where it may cause bronchospasm and wheezing. (Chapter 9 provides a closer look at some of these other allergies and ways to treat them.)

Numerous studies have indicated just how dangerous allergies can be for people with asthma. In one study of people who had died from severe asthma attacks, researchers found that deaths from asthma were more than twice as likely to occur on days when levels of mold spores were at their highest. Other studies have found that children with asthma who are sensitive to mold spores are more likely to have seasonal asthma attacks that occur when high levels of mold spores fill the air.

Researchers do not know what it is about mold spores that can make them so dangerous for people with asthma. It is possible that mold spores, which are much smaller than pollen spores, pass more easily into the lower airway, where they can trigger an asthma attack. Mold spores may also interact with other allergens and environmental air pollution, thus increasing the asthma risk from those substances.

Although this chapter focuses on the relationship between asthma and allergies, it's important to remember that not all asthma is related to allergy and that not all allergies can cause an asthma attack. As we have seen, asthma attacks can be triggered by exposure to nonallergic irritants, such as tobacco smoke, respiratory infections, exercise, cold air, aspirin, air pollution, odors, irritants, and even emotions such as laughing, yelling, crying, and hyperventilating.

DID YOU KNOW...?

Asthma and allergies did not stop Hall of Fame pitcher Bob Gibson from pursuing his dreams. Gibson was one of the fiercest competitors ever to play baseball. His fiery fastball and icy glare menaced major league batters for 17 seasons. During his career Gibson set a host of records, many of which still stand.

Gibson was an outstanding pitcher who won 20 or more games in five separate seasons. But his performance when the pressure was on, in the World Series, is what sets him apart from other pitchers. He holds World Series records for most consecutive games pitched, with 7; for the most strike-outs in one game, with 17; and for the most strike-outs in any single World Series, with 35.

Gibson fought off hitters for the St. Louis Cardinals from 1959 to his retirement in 1975. But the right-hander was fighting off other opponents long before his baseball career began: asthma and allergies.

"I remember having breathing problems all my life," Gibson says. Born in 1935, long before doctors had uncovered many of the secrets about asthma and allergies, Gibson says the first treatment he remembers is his mother rubbing some mentholated ointment on his chest in an attempt to open his constricted airways.

The first time he received specifically designed asthma medications was when he broke into baseball. "When I was growing up, there just wasn't much known about asthma, but by the time I started playing baseball, they had developed some asthma medications, and the team had physicians who cared for me."

Despite the lack of knowledge about asthma and allergies, Gibson says, he never let his condition stop him from pursuing what he wanted. "It's something that you have to overcome and live with. You can't let it get the better of you, and there is no reason for it to hold you back."

Gibson treats his asthma symptoms with inhaled albuterol, an adrenergic drug that relaxes constricted airways. Because his condition is under control, he uses the inhaler only when his wheezing flares up. He takes antihistamines for allergic rhinitis symptoms and gets monthly allergy shots to try to decrease his overactive IgE antibodies. Skin tests have found that Gibson is allergic to grasses, weeds, trees, ragweed pollen, mold spores, house dust mites, and cat and dog dander.

Even in retirement, Gibson doesn't let his asthma and allergies get the better of him. He still throws batting practice during the Cardinals' spring training and is active in educating children with asthma. "These kids have to know that they can do anything they want to do, as long as they take care of their disease," he says.

While both forms of asthma are serious conditions that require proper monitoring and treatment, many doctors feel that allergy-triggered asthma poses the greater problem. Whether you or your family member has allergic or nonallergic asthma, an attack can be triggered by exposure to any of the nonallergic irritants listed above. People with asthma and allergies also are prone to asthma attacks when they encounter any allergy trigger that leads to inflammation and constriction in their airways. Add to this the misery that comes with an allergic reaction, ranging from watery eyes and runny nose to hives and rashes, and you can see that people with both asthma and allergies get a double shot of trouble.

This does not mean that people with asthma and allergies are relegated to lives less fulfilling than those of people without these conditions. On the contrary, these conditions can be controlled, and sufferers can lead normal lives, partaking in virtually whatever activity they wish. To succeed at this, they need to understand their disease, identify their asthma triggers, take steps to avoid these offending substances, and use medications that can dampen their effects.

The link between asthma and allergies starts before birth. Many doctors believe that asthma and allergies are passed on genetically from parents to their children. While some research is beginning to hone in on the elusive gene or genes responsible for asthma or allergies, their exact location remains a mystery. Nonetheless, because the rate of these diseases is higher in children of parents who have asthma or allergies than in children of parents who do not have these diseases, doctors are convinced that these genes exist.

Doctors are also convinced that when they find where on human chromosomes these asthma and allergy genes live, they will find that they are close neighbors. That's because of the strikingly large number of people who have both conditions. The theory is that if you inherit the gene for one condition, you probably will inherit the gene or genes that cause both disorders, since they live so close to each other.

The Airway Link

Allergies can affect people with asthma in a variety of ways. We already have seen how allergens can trigger an asthma attack, and later in this chapter we'll take a closer look at this relationship. The most common allergy is allergic rhinitis. This condition, more commonly known as hay fever, is very closely related to asthma and can lead to a number of problems in people who also have asthma.

Allergic rhinitis is an inflammation of the lining of the nose. In people who have allergic rhinitis, the tissues in the upper airway, especially in the nose and sinuses, become inflamed when exposed to pollen and other allergens. The effects of an inflamed upper airway are all too common to people who sneeze their way through the pollen season. But an inflamed upper airway has important implications for people with asthma.

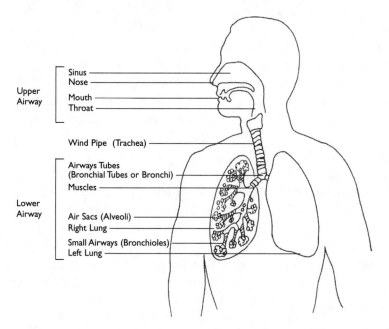

Allergies that affect the upper airway can trigger
an asthma attack in the lower airway.

The nose is a natural air filter. When we breathe through our noses, tiny hairs act to filter out irritating particles before they enter the lower airway. People with allergic rhinitis often have trouble breathing through their noses and are forced to breathe through their mouths instead. This increases the chance that allergic and nonallergic asthma triggers can find their way into the bronchioles of the lungs and, through a variety of chemical reactions, cause airway inflammation leading to the constriction of the airways and increased production of mucus. These processes are what in turn cause the wheezing and coughing commonly associated with asthma.

Looking at the two airways as one continuous pathway, it's easy to see how an allergic response anywhere in this pathway can cause airway inflammation and constriction throughout. That is precisely the case with allergic rhinitis. Doctors now realize that the same allergic reaction that causes the symptoms of hay fever can also trigger an asthma attack. Indeed, as more is learned about these two conditions, doctors increasingly refer to the entire airway rather than making any distinction between the upper and lower parts. If you or someone in your family has asthma and allergies, you should view these diseases as existing hand in hand. And you should think of the airways as one continuous pathway that serves to get needed oxygen to the body.

The IgE Link

As we have seen, allergies depend on an IgE response that causes mast cells to release irritating and inflammatory chemicals that in turn cause airway inflammation and constriction. Doctors can test for levels of IgE in the blood and skin, and indeed, this is one way that they determine if a person has allergies.

Examining levels of IgE antibodies in the blood has also helped reveal the link between asthma and allergies. In one study published by the American Lung Association, doctors found that children born to parents with high IgE levels were more likely to develop asthma. After looking at more than 1,000 children in Tucson, Arizona, doctors found that parents with the highest blood levels of IgE antibodies were most likely to have children with asthma; even those parents with only moderate levels of IgE antibodies were more likely to have children with asthma than those with low IgE levels.

The same study also pointed out the symbiotic relationship between asthma and allergies. Doctors found that children with asthma had far higher levels of IgE antibodies than they would have suspected simply by measuring the levels of IgE in their parents. This seems to indicate that asthma itself, and the inflammation it causes in the airways, can signal the body to overproduce IgE antibodies. This flood of IgE in turn serves to leave people with asthma more prone to the effects of various allergens. Thus, when exposed to allergens in the future, their bodies recognize and react with an overabundance of IgE, triggering allergies and asthma attacks. It is almost as if these conditions could not exist without each other.

Another study published by the American Lung Association found that children who have both asthma and allergies are far less likely to outgrow bouts of wheezing than are children with nonallergy-triggered asthma. This observation has many implications. First, it supports the debunking of the myth that you can outgrow asthma. Since 80 percent of all people with asthma also have allergies, and since people with both conditions tend not to outgrow bouts of wheezing, you can see that the overwhelming majority of people with asthma will have this condition for life.

Second, it is yet more evidence of the link between asthma and allergies. Doctors in this study tested more than 1,000 children in New Zealand for asthma and allergies. They found that children who wheezed at age 9 but had very low levels of IgE were likely to have their wheezing symptoms disappear by age 15. However, the overwhelming majority of children with asthma who had high levels of IgE continued to have asthma attacks. It is possible that children who have asthma symptoms when they are young but do not have high IgE levels grow out of their condition as the size of the airways grows larger and can accommodate more air. Children with asthma who also have allergies, however, are always prone to airway inflammation when their excitable IgE antibodies cause mast cells to release damaging chemicals. This pattern of inflammation is something they never outgrow.

Since everyone has IgE antibodies, it would seem that everyone should suffer from allergies and that everybody with asthma should suffer from allergy-triggered attacks. Of course, this is not the case.

One reason is that the levels of IgE in people with asthma and allergies are far higher than in people who do not suffer from these conditions. When there are too many IgE antibodies living on the surfaces of mast cells, it may be more likely for allergens to become attached to these antibodies, excite them, and in turn cause mast cells to activate. Doctors do not know why people with asthma and allergies may have too many IgE antibodies. It could be that they are born with a genetic system that causes the body to produce too many IgE antibodies—that is, they have inherited this condition from their parents.

Another reason that IgE antibodies do not work their harm on everyone is that people with asthma and allergies have IgE antibodies that are specific for recognizing one or more allergens, including dust mites, pollens, molds, animal fur, certain foods, medications, and others. This process is called sensitization and means that these IgE antibodies have become able to locate and latch onto these allergens. Doctors do not know how or why people become sensitive to certain allergens. Most allergy experts believe that in order to become sensitized to any substance, you must possess the genes that are responsible for turning on the system. People who have these genes are said to be predisposed to developing allergies. Some experts believe that people with a genetic predisposition to develop allergies can become sensitized to certain allergens if they are exposed to them as very young children or if they come into repeated contact with these allergens later in life.

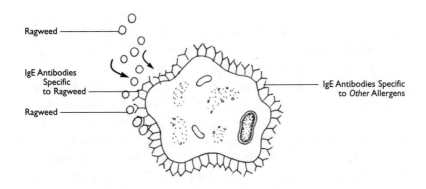

Allergens lock on to receptors on mast cells, causing them to release chemicals that cause an asthma attack.

Finally, people with asthma and allergies may react to allergens because they lack parts of the immune system that turn off an IgE response. Doctors believe there may be at least two parts of the immune system that do not adequately inhibit the effects of IgE in people with allergies and allergy-triggered asthma. Allergy shots are thought to work by boosting the immune system to better inhibit the effects of IgE. (More information about allergy shots is provided in chapter 9.)

Diagnosing Allergies

If you or someone in your family has asthma, you will want to see an asthma specialist. In chapter 2 we outlined the diagnostic workup that your doctor is likely to go through in determining whether you have asthma and how severe the asthma is. Since it is likely that if you have asthma you also have allergies, it is also important to know what allergens might be triggering your asthma.

Allergists have tools at their disposal to identify what substances cause your allergies and which of these substances may trigger an asthma attack. Perhaps the two most common of these tools are a blood test (called RAST) to determine levels of IgE antibodies and skin tests to determine what substances can trigger allergies and allergy-triggered asthma. Skin tests are more sensitive in predicting an allergy than the RAST test and cost less. A blood test and skin tests to determine levels of IgE antibodies can be important tools in identifying allergies. If these tests detect elevated levels of IgE antibodies in the blood, an allergic condition is likely. For some people who also have documented asthma, high levels of IgE in the blood may indicate the need for aggressive use of asthma medications to lower the chance of experiencing severe asthma attacks. Whether you or your family member has asthma, if these tests determine high IgE levels, your doctor will want to perform other tests to confirm these results and determine what substances can trigger an allergic reaction.

When performing skin tests, doctors use diluted liquids made from the actual allergens. Skin tests can check for allergies to various types of pollens, molds, foods, and animal danders. The allergist applies these liquid allergens by pricking the surface of the skin and dropping a tiny amount of the allergen extract into the scratch mark. After 15 to 20 minutes, he or she will check to see if any of the allergens cause a small "mosquito-bite" type of allergic reaction. What the allergist is looking for is a kind of rash or hive that doctors call a wheal. If you have allergies, you have IgE antibodies that recognize and react to any of the substances that cause a wheal. However, only with a careful history taken by the allergist can your doctor decide what substances trigger your disease.

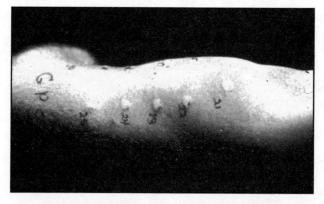

Photo of a skin test for diagnosing allergies and wheal reaction.

After a skin test you will have to wait in the doctor's office for about half an hour to make sure that the reaction is not stronger than expected. Most skin test reactions include swelling and itching around the scratch or puncture. However, more serious allergic reactions can occur. If this happens, the allergist will administer a medication to reverse the reaction. Allergy tests can be slightly uncomfortable, as they cause slight swelling and itching that can last an hour or so. But the knowledge they yield can be powerful. You will know to which substances you are sensitive and which substances may trigger an asthma attack. Armed with this information, you will be able to avoid these substances as much as possible, and you will know when to take asthma and allergy medications to prevent or cut short an attack.

8 / Allergic Rhinitis

YOUR EYES ARE WATERY AND ITCHY, YOUR NOSE RUNNY, ITCHY, and congested. Your throat is scratchy, and you feel like your head is under water. The pressure in your sinuses is causing a throbbing headache. Without warning, you are thrown into uncontrollable fits of sneezing. You can't seem to concentrate. You are distracted from your work, since every time you take the tissue away from your nose it begins running again. While everyone else is looking forward to the start of spring, you worry about the misery the new season will bring. If these symptoms sound familiar, you probably have allergic rhinitis, commonly called hay fever.

An estimated 40 to 50 million Americans suffer from allergies, according to the National Institute of Allergy and Infectious Diseases. Allergic rhinitis, the most common of all allergies, affects an estimated 26 million and was the reason for 7.6 million office visits to physicians in 1992. Allergic rhinitis is primarily an allergy to pollen. Pollen triggers allergic rhinitis symptoms, just as allergens trigger an asthma attack. It stimulates IgE antibodies, causing mast cells to explode and release chemicals that cause airway inflammation. When this inflammation takes place in the upper airway, it produces the misery of allergic rhinitis. But as we saw in chapter 7, inflammation in the upper airway can also trigger cells in the lower airway to react. For people who also have asthma, this can mean the beginnings of an attack.

Allergic Rhinitis and Asthma

If you or someone in your family has both asthma and allergic rhinitis, you are not alone. People with allergic rhinitis are about six times more likely to have asthma than people who do not have the allergy. Up to 58 percent of adults with allergic rhinitis also have asthma, compared with between 3 and 10 percent of people who do not have the allergy. Current bouts of allergic rhinitis appear to be a far greater risk factor for developing asthma than having had the allergy in the past. This furthers the belief that these two conditions operate in tandem. When some allergen affects one of these conditions, it is possible that both will flare up.

If you or someone in your family has allergic rhinitis but has not had problems with asthma, you may not be out of the woods. People with allergic rhinitis are more likely to develop asthma at some point in their life than are people who do not have the allergy. In one study of 738 college students tested for allergic rhinitis, doctors found that those who had the allergy but did not have asthma were more likely to go on to develop asthma than were students who did not have allergic rhinitis. About 10 percent of students who had allergic rhinitis in 1963 developed asthma within the following 23 years, compared to less than 4 percent of students who did not have the allergy that year.

Because of the profound link between allergic rhinitis and asthma, some researchers have found that allergy shots aimed at boosting the immune system may also reduce asthma in some people. Allergy shots, also known as immunotherapy, are a treatment for allergies. The therapy consists of injecting very small amounts of known allergens in increasing doses so that the immune system can fight the allergic reaction. The amounts of allergens in the injections are usually too small to cause an allergic reaction, but occasionally they do cause a reaction, so care and caution must be taken. Allergy shots are thought to work by stimulating parts of the immune system to recognize the offending allergens and shut off the allergic response. Allergy shots for allergic rhinitis are discussed in greater detail later in this chapter.

In one study by doctors at Johns Hopkins University School of Medicine, allergy shots made with tiny amounts of ragweed pollen lessened asthma symptoms. The doctors tried the therapy on 77 people whose asthma was triggered during ragweed season. After giving the shots every week for two full allergy seasons, they found that people with asthma triggered by ragweed pollen had better peak expiratory flow measurements year-round. They also found that those who received the injections were less likely to have a drop in their peak flow tests during ragweed season than were people with asthma who did not receive the shots. When the people in the study were asked how they felt, those who received the allergy shots reported a 40 percent drop in asthma attacks.

Studies like these point out the importance of allergic rhinitis in asthma. In chapter 7 we saw how an allergy that affects any part of the airways can trigger an asthma attack. Allergic rhinitis, being the most common allergy, affects many people with asthma and may be linked to this breathing condition over time. If you or someone in your family has asthma and allergic rhinitis, you must learn to control both of these conditions. Therapies for treating allergies are discussed later in this chapter. These therapies, combined with an asthma control plan, can reduce the chance of asthma and allergy attacks.

"Maria"

Maria was 18 months old in the middle of 1996 when her mother, Teresa, took her to the doctor for a nagging cough. The first words out of the pediatrician's mouth were "'How long has this child been wheezing?'" Teresa recalls. "The first thing I thought was 'What a bad parent I must be not even being able to recognize that my daughter was wheezing.' Then I realized I didn't know what wheezing was."

The doctor told Teresa that wheezing was a symptom of asthma and, although he wanted to do more tests, he was relatively certain that Maria had asthma. "I wanted to cry," Teresa says. "My perfectly healthy baby had asthma, and everyone knows that asthma is some psychosomatic disease caused by the mother." But the doctor told Teresa her beliefs about asthma could not be further from the truth. "I learned that asthma is a real disease, that it is not psychosomatic, and that it has nothing to do with parenting skills," she says.

Maria was diagnosed with moderate asthma. The doctor prescribed a regimen of inhaled cromolyn, to be delivered through a nebulizer with a face mask three times a day. He also prescribed a liquid beta-adrenergic drug that Teresa was to give her daughter when she was wheezing. But there was more. The doctor told Teresa that it was probable that Maria was allergic to the family dog. Although the medications would help, unless Maria's exposure to the dog was reduced, her asthma would keep flaring up. "It was a tough decision, because my husband and I had had the dog for a number of years, but when we were told that our little girl was allergic, we decided the best thing was to give the dog to a friend," Teresa says.

Managing Maria's asthma is a continual learning process for Teresa and her husband. They understand that Maria will probably never outgrow her asthma, but they are committed to making sure she leads a normal life. As Maria gets older, Teresa says she plans to teach her how to use the nebulizer and later a pocket-sized inhaler so she can develop a sense of independence. "My husband and I now know about asthma and what needs to be done. It took a lot of reading and listening, but we understand that this is a chronic disease, that we need to manage it, but that there is no reason it should hold Maria back," she says. ❑

What Is Rhinitis?

Allergic rhinitis is one of a number of rhinitis disorders. The word *rhinitis* means inflammation of the lining of the nose. When allergies cause this inflammation, the condition is called allergic rhinitis. Other rhinitis disorders include infectious rhinitis (another name for the common cold and other upper-airway infections) and chronic rhinitis. People with chronic rhinitis have constantly inflamed membranes in their nose and sinuses. Chronic rhinitis can stem from allergic rhinitis in people who are sensitive to many allergens in the air. In one study of 200 people who had undergone surgery to correct the inflammation causing their chronic rhinitis, doctors found that nearly 28 percent also had allergies. Chronic rhinitis does not have to be linked to allergies; it can also be linked to other disorders in the upper airways, such as nasal polyps, sinusitis, or ear infections. The same study found that more than half of the people with chronic rhinitis had nasal polyps, small growths inside the nose and sinuses that can impede breathing.

All forms of rhinitis are important, especially among people with asthma. As we have seen, any condition that prohibits an asthma sufferer from breathing through the natural air filters in the nose can serve to trigger an attack by allowing increased amounts of asthma triggers and cooler, drier air into the lower airways. When asthma is present, allergic rhinitis is the most important of these rhinitis disorders. Indeed, people with allergic rhinitis are three to five times more likely to have asthma than people with other types of rhinitis.

Types of Allergic Rhinitis

Allergic rhinitis falls into two categories: seasonal and perennial. Seasonal allergic rhinitis is more commonly known as hay fever, although sufferers are not necessarily allergic to hay, nor do they have a fever. Hay fever got its name because hay is harvested early in the farming season when ragweed pollen abounds. It used to be assumed that hay dust caused the sneezing. People with seasonal allergic rhinitis have a seasonal pattern to their symptoms. As discussed in chapter 6, this pattern is related to the times during which various pollens or mold spores are carried on the wind.

The hay fever season generally starts in February or March, depending on the area of the country. This coincides with the appearance of the first tree pollens. Beginning in early May and lasting through July, grass pollens take over. Weeds begin to bloom around the beginning of July and are followed by the infamous ragweed plant, which comes into bloom around mid-August to late September, reaching a peak between late August and mid-September. Even after the plant has stopped producing pollen, this potent pollen can continue to cause hay fever misery lasting until the pollen grains are killed during the first frost.

Mold spores can ignite IgE reactions at any time of the year, but levels of the spores tend to peak in the spring and fall in most of the country. In Southern states, mold spores are present year-round.

Flowering plants are less of a problem for people with asthma and allergies because these flowers tend to have large, waxy pollens that are carried from one plant to the next by bees. The pollen from these plants does not have as much of a chance to become airborne and inhaled by people with asthma and allergies. However, chrysanthemums and marigolds can cross-react with ragweed pollens and cause people to be miserable.

If you or a family member has asthma or allergies, you may want to plan your garden to take advantage of as many low-allergy plants as possible. Start by choosing showier flowering plants that are pollinated by bees. This will reduce the levels of airborne pollen in your garden. You should also avoid as much as possible some of the worst pollen producers. These include trees such as oak, western red cedar, elm, birch, ash, hickory, poplar, sycamore, maple, cypress, and walnut; grasses such as timothy, Bermuda, orchard, sweet vernal, red top, and bluegrass; and weeds such as ragweed, sagebrush, pigweed, tumbleweed, Russian thistle, and cockleweed. People with asthma and allergies should also be careful about the yard work they perform. Raking leaves and cutting grass can kick up a lot of pollen. If you want to do yard work, try taking an antihistamine about 30 minutes ahead of time. You may also want to use a particle mask and sunglasses when working in the yard to limit the amount of pollen inhaled or blown into the eyes.

Perennial allergic rhinitis causes symptoms similar to hay fever but is not connected to the time of year. The symptoms can be triggered by nonseasonal allergens such as dust mites, animal danders, wool, feathers, and indoor and outdoor mold spores, as well as by seasonal pollen.

Recognizing Allergic Rhinitis

You should suspect seasonal or perennial allergic rhinitis if you or a family member suffers from a recurring pattern of symptoms each spring, summer, or fall, or if these symptoms occur year-round but appear to be linked to exposure to some allergens. The most common symptoms in allergic rhinitis include:

- violent, prolonged sneezing spells
- watery, clear nasal discharge
- nasal congestion, nose itching or rubbing
- reduction in the sense of smell
- breathing through the mouth
- constant clearing of the throat
- itching, tearing eyes
- itching in the eyes, mouth, and throat

Allergies and colds share many symptoms. But the achiness and fever that accompany a cold rarely occur with an allergy. And colds seldom cause itching, whereas allergies produce widespread itching in the eyes, nose, and throat. You should suspect allergic rhinitis if you or a family member has cold symptoms that do not seem to clear up. Persistent cold symptoms may indicate allergic rhinitis. The table in this chapter compares the symptoms in allergic rhinitis with those of most colds and respiratory infections. Use it when trying to determine if the symptoms you or your family member is experiencing may signal allergic rhinitis.

How to Distinguish Hay Fever from a Cold

Symptom	Allergic Rhinitis	Common Cold, Flu, or Respiratory Infection
Nasal discharge	Thin, watery, clear	Thick, yellow to green in color
Fever	None	Occasionally, low-grade
Itching	In ears, nose, and throat	Rare
Sneezing	Often occurring in violent, prolonged spells	Occasional
Duration	Weeks to months	7 to 10 days

Spotting allergic rhinitis in children requires special attention. Children who suffer from hay fever are especially prone to be moody, listless, and irritable because they feel miserable. Parents need to watch for these behavioral symptoms as possible indications that allergies have arrived. They can then begin using medications to help clear their children's symptoms and perhaps their mood.

Treating Allergic Rhinitis

If you or someone in your family has allergic rhinitis, you'll want it treated. This condition can cause such misery during the pollen season that people with allergies often go to great extremes to relieve their suffering. For a person with asthma, treating allergic rhinitis is doubly important. As we have seen, hay fever flares can trigger an asthma attack. They can also eliminate the use of the natural air-filtering mechanisms in the nose, leaving people with asthma more apt to inhale asthma triggers through their mouths. Properly controlled allergic rhinitis can take the misery out of the pollen season and help prevent many asthma attacks.

There are six basic options for treating allergic rhinitis. The following paragraphs describe these therapies and suggest how they may fit into your allergy and asthma maintenance plan.

Antihistamines work by mopping up excess amounts of histamine, one of the chemicals released by mast cells. Histamine causes airways to become irritated and inflamed, and produces many of the symptoms felt during an allergy attack, including sneezing and itching. Because older types of antihistamine caused drowsiness, they were inconvenient to take during the day. Newer, nonsedating antihistamines have little or no drowsiness side effect and are quite effective.

Decongestants are medications that open clogged nasal passages. They are often given in conjunction with antihistamines. Some preparations contain both an antihistamine and a decongestant.

Steroid nasal sprays can be miniature metered-dose sprays or misting devices. The medication is inhaled into each nostril and works by reducing inflammation in the nasal passages and sinuses.

Cromolyn comes in nasal inhalers for allergies, just as it does in oral inhalers for asthma. This drug works by reducing inflammation in the nasal passages and by dampening the effects of some allergens, as well as by stabilizing mast cells to prevent them from releasing their irritating chemicals.

Immunotherapy, or allergy shots, works by stimulating parts of the immune system to decrease levels of IgE antibodies. The injections must be given regularly and for prolonged periods. Researchers are investigating whether immunotherapy can be given in nasal sprays. This form of treatment is still experimental but holds the promise of short-circuiting the allergic response without the discomfort of allergy shots.

Avoidance is the one form of treatment that every person with allergies should try. By reducing your exposure to pollen and molds, you can reduce many allergy attacks and the amount of medication needed to control your symptoms. Avoidance comes with no side effects and can be readily employed by anybody with allergic rhinitis. Avoidance should begin by recognizing which pollens cause your allergic rhinitis symptoms. The most common sources of offending pollen are listed earlier in this chapter, under "Types of Allergic Rhinitis."

By following the tips in chapter 6 for controlling asthma and allergy triggers, you can significantly reduce the number of times you or your family member will suffer from hay fever. Remember that if you have allergic rhinitis, you can take part in virtually any activity you wish; it is just a matter of planning and control. You can exercise, garden, and take part in outdoor activities by following the simple steps outlined in chapter 6.

Avoidance Measures for Allergic Rhinitis

- Use an air conditioner to filter the air when possible.
- Stretch your time indoors to reduce time spent outside.
- Wash pollen off your body and hair after exercising.
- Wear a mask and sunglasses when gardening or doing yard work.

Antihistamines

There are dozens of antihistamine drugs available to treat allergic rhinitis. These compounds work by blocking the effects of histamine, the chemical responsible for causing many allergy symptoms. Antihistamines accomplish this by blocking areas on cells to which histamine attaches. If histamine is prevented from reaching these areas, the chemical cannot cause the sneezing, itchy eyes, and runny nose that are common in people with hay fever. When used over time, antihistamines also reduce the amount of histamine released by stimulated mast cells.

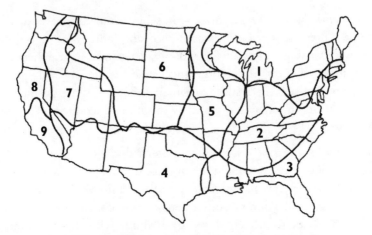

When do allergy causing pollens bloom in your backyard?

Area	Ragweed	Trees	Grasses
1	July-September	February-June	May-November
2	August-September	March-June	June-November
3	August-October	April-June	May-September
4	July-October	March-July	May-November
5	August-October	March-June	May-October
6	June-November	January-July	April-November
7	June-September	January-April	April-October
8	June-November	March-June	May-October
9	August-September	March-June	May-August

It is important to remember that antihistamines work best before histamine is released by mast cells. Therefore it is advisable to take antihistamines before an allergic reaction begins. These drugs also work better when they are taken on a regular basis. Doctors often prescribe antihistamines to be used regularly throughout the height of the pollen season.

Antihistamines are either sedating or nonsedating. Many older, sedating antihistamines are available over-the-counter. Some over-the-counter cold remedies also contain sedating antihistamines. These medications, while quite effective in many people with allergic rhinitis, can make users very sleepy and drowsy. They can also cause dry mouth. Newer antihistamines, available only through prescription, cause these side effects to a much lesser degree.

At one time it was thought that antihistamines should not be mixed with asthma medications because the combination was thought to lead to potentially serious side effects. In fact, many products still carry a warning that the drug not be taken by people with asthma. Most asthma and allergy experts now agree that antihistamines can be taken by people with asthma and indeed be part of the care plan of someone who has both asthma and allergies.

Antihistamines

Sedating Antihistamines	
Generic Name	*Brand Name*
clemastine fumarate	Tavist
diphenhydramine	Benadryl
chlorpheniramine	Allerest
dexbrompheniramine	Drixoral
Less Sedating Antihistamines	
Generic Name	*Brand Name*
cetirizine	Zyrtec
Nonsedating Antihistamines	
Generic Name	*Brand Name*
astemizole	Hismanal
loratadine	Claritin
fexofenadine	Allegra

Effects: Antihistamines dry out membranes in the nose and sinuses and subdue bouts of sneezing and itchy, watery eyes.

Possible side effects: Drowsiness, sleepiness, restlessness, and dry mouth in older preparations. Few side effects in newer, nonsedating antihistamines. Nonsedating antihistamines have been linked to a rare occurrence of abnormal heartbeat in people who also were taking certain antibiotic and antifungal medications. If you are taking an antibiotic, antifungal, or ulcer medication drug, tell your doctor. He or she will determine if the medication you are taking can interact with these nonsedating antihistamines.

Time considerations: Antihistamines work best when taken before an allergic reaction begins and when taken regularly. Older, sedating antihistamines may work in about 30 minutes, while newer, nonsedating antihistamines may take up to one hour to a few days to work.

Doses: The dose of an antihistamine depends on which product is being used.

Comments: If you start taking an antihistamine at the beginning of the pollen season, the chances are good that you will reduce allergy symptoms. Take precautions when using an over-the-counter cold remedy, cough syrup, or other medication on top of your prescribed antihistamine, since many of these remedies contain antihistamines and you could significantly increase the amount of the drug you are taking. Be sure to carefully read the ingredients on any medication purchased over-the-counter to know just what you are taking.

Decongestants

As many antihistamines as there are stocked on the shelves of pharmacies, there are at least that many decongestants. These medications work to dry up tissues in the nasal passages and to reduce swollen membranes in the nose. Decongestants come in liquids, pills, sprays, and nose drops. Most are sold over-the-counter. Decongestants often are combined with an antihistamine in a single preparation.

Some Decongestants

Generic Name	Brand Names
oxymetazoline	Afrin
pseudoephedrine	Sudafed, Afrinol
phenylephrine	Coricidin, Neo-Synephrine

Among decongestants, the nasal sprays and drops are most often used and abused. You should not use nasal decongestant sprays or drops for more than 5 days in a row. After about 4 to 5 days, the time that these nasal sprays and drops control your symptoms decreases, so the medication must be used more often to provide relief. Eventually a phenomenon known as the rebound effect can occur, in which the decongestant nasal spray or drops, after the initial useful effect, actually begin to cause the nasal congestion they were designed to inhibit. At the same time the user begins using the product more often and in greater amounts but gets less and less relief. The only way to break the cycle is to stop using the sprays or drops and to see your doctor for more appropriate medications.

Effects: Decongestants dry up nasal tissues and reduce inflammation in the nasal passages.

Some Antihistamine/Decongestant Preparations

Sedating Agents		
Brand Name	*Antihistamine*	*Decongestant*
Actifed	triprolidine	pseudoephedrine
Contact	chlorpheniramine	phenylpropanolamine
Dimetapp	brompheniramine	phenylephrine
Dristan	chlorpheniramine	phenylephrine
Sudafed-Plus	chlorpheniramine	pseudoephedrine
Nonsedating Agents		
Brand Name	*Antihistamine*	*Decongestant*
Claritin-D	loratadine	pseudoephedrine

Side effects: These drugs can cause sleeplessness, nervousness, jitteriness, racing heartbeat, and rapid pulse. If you have high blood pressure, a heart condition, thyroid disease, diabetes, glaucoma, or prostate problems, you should talk to your doctor before taking decongestants.

Time considerations: Liquid and pill decongestants work in about 30 minutes. Nasal sprays and drops work within minutes but must not be used for more than 5 days in a row because of the rebound effect.

Doses: As with antihistamines, the dose of a decongestant depends on the product being used.

Comments: Overuse of decongestants can dry out nasal passages too much. Never use a decongestant nasal spray or drops for more than 5 days in a row.

Steroid Nasal Sprays

Steroids are potent anti–inflammatory drugs that are highly effective in decreasing the inflammation in the nasal passages of people with allergic rhinitis. When used for allergic rhinitis, steroids come in miniature metered–dose inhalers and pump spray misters for use directly in the nose. The metered–dose inhalers work much like asthma inhalers, in that a propellant forces a mist of the medication out through a tiny opening that fits inside the nostril. Pump spray misters work like over-the-counter nasal decongestant sprays. The tip must be depressed rapidly, forcing a fine mist of the medication through the nose piece. Refer to the table on page 114 for tips on using nasal inhalers.

Steroid Nasal Inhalers

Generic Name	Brand Names
beclomethasone	Beconase, Vancenase
budesonide	Rhinocort
flunisolide	Nasalide, Nasarel
triamcinolone	Nasacort
fluticasone	Flonase

These inhalers are most effective if you or your family member with allergic rhinitis starts using them about a week before the allergy season starts. That's because, as with steroid inhalers for asthma, it takes about a week for these drugs to start working to reduce the underlying inflammation in the nasal passages. Steroid nasal inhalers may be given to anyone with significant allergic rhinitis symptoms. The Food and Drug Administration has cleared the way for children age 6 and older to use some of these inhalers. Check with your doctor if your child is under 6 years of age.

Effects: Steroid nasal sprays reduce the underlying inflammation in the nasal passages of people with allergic rhinitis. They work in much the same way that steroid inhalers for asthma work. By reducing this inflammation, the nasal passages open more clearly and allow more air to be taken in through the natural air filters in the nose.

Side effects: Sneezing, dryness or a burning sensation in the nostrils, and a bad taste in the mouth. These sprays may cause mild irritation of the tissues in the nose.

Time considerations: Steroid nasal inhalers may take up to 2 weeks before they begin to reduce inflammation in the nasal passages. You should talk to your doctor about these drugs before the allergy season starts in your area. They work best to prevent the symptoms of allergic rhinitis when begun at least a week before the start of the pollen season.

Doses: Your doctor will determine the dose that is best for the symptoms you or your family member suffers from. Generally, a dose of 2 puffs in each nostril 2 to 4 times a day is recommended. Children between ages 6 to 12 typically receive 1 puff in each nostril 2 to 3 times a day.

Comments: For steroid nasal inhalers to work, the medication must reach deep in the back tissues of the nasal passages. If you or your family member with allergic rhinitis has a very runny or stuffy nose, the medication may not reach the tissues it needs to. You should try blowing your nose before using these sprays. If the nose is too congested to clear, your doctor may recommend another drug to clear this congestion for the first few days that you use a steroid inhaler. Remember that these drugs work best when begun about a week before the allergy season starts.

Cromolyn

Cromolyn nasal spray works to reduce nasal inflammation without the use of steroids. This drug may also stabilize mast cells, thus helping to prevent them from exploding and releasing their inflammatory chemicals. Cromolyn is a very effective drug for allergic rhinitis symptoms and has few side effects. Unfortunately, as with asthma, this drug does not work in all people with allergic rhinitis.

One form of cromolyn nasal spray, called Nasalcrom, is sold in the United States. It has been approved by the Food and Drug Administration for use in children as young as 6 years of age. Ask your doctor if this drug is appropriate for your child. As with steroid nasal sprays, this drug works best when started before the allergy season begins. It can take as long as two weeks before the effect of this drug on reducing nasal inflammation and the allergic response is seen.

Effects: Cromolyn reduces inflammation in the nasal passages and may help subdue the allergic reaction.

Side effects: Sneezing, dry or burning feeling in the nostrils, and bad taste in the mouth.

Time considerations: Cromolyn may take up to 2 weeks to work to reduce inflammation and dampen the allergic response. It is best to start taking this drug about 2 weeks before the allergy season begins.

Doses: In adults, 2 puffs in each nostril 2 to 4 times a day. Children ages 6 to 12 generally receive 1 puff in each nostril 2 to 4 times a day.

Comments: Cromolyn nasal spray is especially effective in mild to moderate allergic rhinitis. Some adults get good results from the drug in preventing hay fever symptoms. Cromolyn does not relieve symptoms once they are present; it is used as a drug to prevent symptoms from appearing. A related product called nedocromil, or Tilade, is sometimes used when other medications and avoidance techniques have failed to control allergies.

TIPS FOR USING A NASAL INHALER

➤ Shake the product well before using.

➤ Try clearing nose by blowing into a tissue.

➤ Tip head back slightly and insert the tip of the nose piece in one nostril.

➤ Press the canister if using a metered-dose inhaler, or rapidly squeeze the pump actuator on pump mister devices.

➤ Inhale fully as you press or squeeze the inhaler.

➤ Hold breath for a few seconds.

➤ Breathe out and repeat procedure in other nostril.

➤ If directed to use 2 puffs in each nostril, wait 2 to 5 minutes before repeating the procedure.

If using a nasal inhaler for children, help by holding the inhaler in the child's nostril and pressing or squeezing the device for the child. If the child is very young and has trouble inhaling at precisely the right time, hold the inhaler in his or her nostril for a few seconds after pressing the inhaler to prevent the medication from leaving the nostril immediately.

Immunotherapy

Immunotherapy, or desensitization therapy, is what is commonly known as allergy shots. When these injections are given regularly, they can help decrease levels of excited IgE antibodies. Immunotherapy consists of a program in which people with allergies are given injections containing very tiny amounts of the allergens to which they are allergic. The injections may be given as often as daily in the beginning, decreasing to once or twice a month. With each visit, people receiving allergy shots receive a slightly higher dose of the allergens until a maintenance level is reached. Generally, the injections are given for 3 to 5 years.

Immunotherapy causes the body to become less sensitive to the allergen or allergens to which a person is allergic. Doctors are not completely sure how this works. But they have some theories based on observations of people who have received the injections. People who have undergone treatments with allergy shots have higher levels of specific IgE-blocking antibodies and lower levels of allergy-causing IgE than they had before receiving the shots. Based on these observations, doctors think that the shots work by preventing IgE antibodies from locking up with allergens. Thus the IgE antibodies do not become excited and cannot cause mast cells to release the chemicals that cause airway inflammation.

In immunotherapy doctors use what are called extracts of allergens. These are tiny amounts of the offending allergens in a liquid solution. Allergen extracts are available for a variety of allergens, including the pollen of many trees, grasses and weeds, molds, dust mites, and animal allergens. Immunotherapy generally is not used to treat people who are allergic to foods, wool, and feathers. Your allergist will determine which extracts to use after taking a detailed history of your allergy symptoms and comparing it with the results of your skin tests. This is done after performing the skin tests discussed in chapter 7.

Immunotherapy can be very effective for people with allergic rhinitis. Experience has shown that allergy shots can provide significant relief in four out of every five people with allergies to grasses and ragweed. The therapy is also effective for people with allergies to tree pollens and dust mites. Less is known about the effectiveness of the shots in relieving allergies to molds. The therapy may be most effective for people who have allergies to only a few different types of pollen or dust mites. When extracts from numerous different trees, grasses, and weeds must be mixed together, each allergen dilutes the other and the effectiveness may decline. In the case of allergies to some pollens, shots that desensitize a person to the pollen of one tree or grass may protect him or her from reactions to plants that are close relatives.

Allergy shots have some drawbacks. They are inconvenient. People with allergies must visit their allergist often in the beginning and at least once a month afterward for up to 5 years. The shots also take time to work. In the beginning you may notice that your allergy symptoms are not as severe, but it may take until the next allergy season before you notice a reduction in the number of times you suffer from hay fever symptoms. And there are some side effects to the injections. Many patients develop swelling at the site of the injection. If this swelling is large, antihistamines or ice may be needed to bring it down. Less common are systemic reactions to the shots, which include sneezing, watery nasal discharge, itchy eyes, swelling in the throat, wheezing or tightness in the chest, dizziness, or even unconsciousness. Systemic side effects occur in about 1 out of every 200 to 500 injections. Because they can be severe, you must wait in your doctor's office for about 30 minutes after the injections so that he or she can be sure the reactions will not occur. Deaths have also occurred from allergy shots, but fortunately this is very rare. Allergy shots are usually safe when administered under the supervision of a specialist who is equipped to treat all the possible reactions that can occur.

To get around the side effects and inconvenience of immunotherapy injections, some doctors are trying to develop a way to administer the therapy in a nasal spray. In a study published by the American Lung Association, doctors in Italy found that nasal immunotherapy may work in people who are allergic to pollens and dust mites. The doctors tested the nasal immunotherapy in a group of 20 people with allergic rhinitis triggered by a specific pollen known as Parietaria. People with allergies began using the nasal spray, which consisted of a dry powder inhaled through a special nasal device, six months before the allergy season began. The people in the study received increasing doses of the allergen extracts twice a week for the first two weeks and then received the same dose once a week for the remainder of the study. The doctors found that people with allergies who used the nasal immunotherapy inhaler had fewer allergy symptoms (including sneezing, itching, runny nose, coughing, and asthma attacks). Nasal immunotherapy is still experimental, but one day people with allergies may be able to use this approach without having to go for daily, weekly, or monthly allergy shots.

Immunotherapy is not for everyone. Whether you or your family member with allergies can be helped by allergy shots depends on what types of allergies are present and how severe they are. Your doctor will decide if immunotherapy is an option. If he or she decides that immunotherapy can help, and if you stick with the program of injections, it can provide significant relief from hay fever suffering.

9 / Other Allergies

ALTHOUGH HAY FEVER—THE ALLERGIC REACTION TO POLLEN and mold spores—is the most common allergy, numerous other substances can trigger the body to launch into an allergic reaction. These substances, or allergens, can be present in certain medications, foods, insect venom, or plant secretions, causing allergic reactions ranging from skin rashes and hives to stomach upset to a potentially fatal reaction known as anaphylaxis. While these other allergies are far less common than hay fever, and their ability to trigger asthma attacks much more rare, they nonetheless represent an important aspect of allergies and asthma.

Nearly 50 million Americans suffer from allergies of one sort or another. As noted in chapter 8, the overwhelming majority of these people are affected by allergic rhinitis, or hay fever. But allergies can also result from other substances that can be introduced into the body through the mouth or by contact with the skin or eyes. This chapter will discuss some of these other types of allergies, how they affect the body, what can trigger these reactions, and how they can be treated. It is important to note that allergies other than hay fever are not common. It is also important to understand that other than anaphylaxis, which is known to cause bronchospasm and severe asthma attacks, the link between these other allergies and asthma is much less clear than the association between asthma and hay fever.

Allergies, whether hay fever or other types of reactions, are the body's response to substances that are perceived as a threat. The allergic reaction is the result of the body's immune defense system racing to counter the effects of any invader. It is the immune system's job to protect the body from substances that can harm it, such as bacteria, viruses, or other foreign substances. When the immune system targets substances that generally pose no threat, the reaction is known as an allergy.

As discussed in earlier chapters, the most important part of the allergic immune system is the IgE antibody, which people with allergies tend to overproduce. When stimulated, IgE antibodies, which are attached to the surface of mast cells, cause the mast cells to release chemicals that in turn cause and amplify inflammation. Chief among these mast cell chemicals is histamine. When histamine is released in the lower respiratory tree, the effect is bronchospasm, with symptoms such as wheezing, coughing, and shortness of breath. In the upper respiratory tree, histamine can lead to the misery of hay fever, including runny nose, teary eyes, nasal itching, and sneezing.

Other allergies work in the body in the same manner as the allergens that trigger asthma attacks and hay fever. When allergens are taken in by the mouth, histamine may be released in the stomach and digestive tract, where it can cause stomach cramps and diarrhea, or in the skin, where it can cause hives and other rashes. Occasionally an allergen may affect the entire body, causing a potentially fatal reaction known as anaphylaxis. During this type of allergic reaction, all organs related to the immune system may react and cause this potentially fatal condition.

The Anaphylactic Reaction

Deaths from anaphylaxis are rare. The federal government estimates that about 1 of every 100 people is at risk for a serious anaphylactic reaction at some time during his or her life. Because not all these reactions are potentially life-threatening, and because medications can reverse an anaphylactic reaction, few people die from the condition. Deaths from two of the major causes of anaphylactic reactions, injections of the antibiotic penicillin and the stings of insects—bees, wasps, hornets, yellow jackets, or fire ants—are better defined. As many as 1 out of every 7.5 million penicillin injections can cause death from anaphylaxis, while the risk of systemic reactions from certain insect stings may range from 0.4 to 4.0 percent of the general population.

During an anaphylactic allergic reaction, massive amounts of histamine and other chemicals that cause inflammation are released from mast cells throughout the body. The massive release of mast cell chemicals causes blood vessels throughout the body to dilate, thus lowering blood pressure and slowing the pulse. Air passages can narrow and impede breathing. Symptoms of an anaphylactic reaction include headache, nausea and vomiting, sneezing and coughing, stomach cramps, hives, swelling of the lips and joints, diarrhea, shortness of breath and wheezing, low blood pressure, convulsions, and loss of consciousness.

Drugs are the leading cause of anaphylactic reactions. The most common drugs that can cause anaphylaxis are antibiotics, aspirin and related compounds, certain seizure medications, muscle relaxants, and blood and blood products. Foods can also cause anaphylaxis, with the most common being milk, eggs, shellfish, nuts, and peanuts. Even some food additives have been implicated in causing anaphylaxis. Sulfites, which are used to preserve dried fruits and vegetables, potato products, and pickles and also are contained in some wines, may be a culprit. Because of this possible link, the Food and Drug Administration has banned sulfites from fresh fruits and vegetables and has mandated that foods containing more than 10 parts of sulfites per million be labeled.

Doctors cannot predict whether your allergies leave you at risk for an anaphylactic reaction. The skin and RAST tests discussed in chapter 7 can determine which substances may cause you to have an allergic response. There is no way, however, to know if exposure to these allergens will trigger a typical allergic reaction or an anaphylactic reaction. Doctors do know that if you have had an anaphylactic reaction, you are likely to have a similar reaction when exposed to the allergen in the future. If you encounter a reaction that comes with the symptoms typically associated with anaphylaxis, your doctor can take a blood sample to look for a chemical called tryptase, which is elevated for about four hours after the reaction and can confirm that your attack was this very serious and severe allergy.

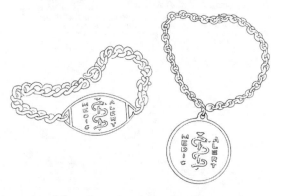

People at risk for a life-threatening allergic reaction called anaphylaxis should wear a Medic Alert bracelet or necklace.

If you have a history of allergies to some of the substances typically associated with anaphylaxis, and skin or RAST tests confirm these allergies, your doctor will probably recommend that you wear a Medic Alert tag. These tags, which can be worn as bracelets, necklaces, or anklets, list the substances to which you are allergic so that emergency medical technicians and doctors will avoid giving you any medications or substances that can trigger your allergies. (See the Asthma and Allergy Resources on page 215 to find out how to obtain a Medic Alert bracelet or necklace.)

Your doctor may also recommend that you carry injectable epinephrine to take at the very first signs of an allergy attack. This medication, which comes in a kit, quickly reverses the allergic reaction. If you are at risk of a repeated anaphylactic reaction, it is extremely important that you carry your kit at all times and know how to use it. An anaphylactic reaction can occur very quickly, leaving little time to seek medical attention. Further, if you encounter a possible anaphylactic allergen when away from medical care, such as while hiking, you need to treat it immediately, at the first sign of a reaction. Do not wait to see if you proceed to develop other symptoms. You cannot know how severe your reaction will become, so it is very important to begin therapy as soon as possible. If you have allergies and are at risk of anaphylaxis, ask your doctor to train you in using an epinephrine injection kit. The three most common kits are sold under the names Ana-Kit, EpiPen, and EpiPen EZ.

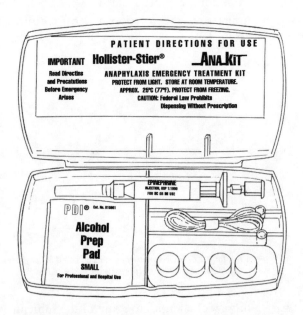

An anaphylaxis emergency kit can reverse the potentially life-threatening reaction.

HOW TO PREPARE FOR AN ANAPHYLACTIC REACTION

1. Carry a supply of epinephrine, available with a doctor's prescription as an EpiPen, Ana-Kit, or EpiPen EZ, at all times.

2. Keep an epinephrine kit in several places, including your car and workplace and, if your child is allergic, at his or her school and with the baby-sitter.

3. Inspect the epinephrine kit and replace it if it has become discolored or has reached the expiration date.

4. Have your doctor teach you, and then you teach other family members, how to use the kit.

5. Have the family member with allergies wear a Medic Alert bracelet or necklace noting the allergy, in case of unconsciousness during a severe attack.

Skin Allergies

Hay fever, while the most common allergy, is only one of a number of related allergic conditions. Chief among these other types of allergies is a condition known as atopic (allergic) dermatitis, or atopic eczema. Eczema is a chronic condition that may begin in early childhood and cause itchy skin rashes. In fact, the itching is the most troublesome symptom of atopic eczema and occurs before the rash develops. The condition is often known as the "itch that rashes." As many as 2 percent of Americans suffer from the condition, though it is more common in people who also have asthma, hay fever, or other allergies. When eczema is the result of an allergic reaction, the condition is called allergic eczema.

Allergic eczema can cause a rash almost anywhere on the body, but it is particularly common on skin folds, such as inside the elbows and behind the knees. The rash takes the form of dry, flaky skin patches that are very itchy and inflamed. Allergic eczema can be caused by many types of allergens, including foods and house dust mites, but doctors do not believe the condition can be caused by other inhaled allergens. A related condition, known as allergic contact dermatitis, results when the skin is directly exposed to some irritating substance, such as poison ivy.

Thousands of chemicals and other substances can cause allergic contact dermatitis, but the most common are poison ivy, the metal

---

ALLERGENS THAT COMMONLY CAUSE ALLERGIC CONTACT DERMATITIS

Plants
    Poison ivy
    Poison oak
    Poison sumac
Metals
    Nickel and chrome—contained in costume jewelry
    Mercury—found in some contact lens solutions
Cosmetics and hair dyes
Medicated creams containing neomycin or penicillin

---

nickel, and certain cosmetics. Poison ivy belongs to a family of plants that includes poison oak and sumac. The allergic reaction is caused by a plant resin called urushiol, which can get on the skin and lead to the well-known itchy poison ivy rash. This resin is so sticky that it can remain on clothes and tools and cause a reaction when touched at some later time. If you have come into contact with poison ivy or other poisonous plants, you should wash all exposed clothing and shoes with hot water and soap.

The rash from poisonous plants is somewhat different from that of typical atopic eczema. The rash starts with a blister-like lesion that is intensely itchy and inflamed. It can take as long as 96 hours after exposure to a poisonous plant before the rash appears. The area of the body that has had the greatest exposure to the plant is the area that will develop the rash first.

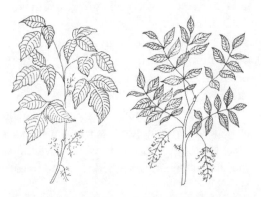

Some plants, such as poison ivy (left) and poison sumac (right), cause a blistering allergic skin reaction.

Allergic contact dermatitis can be caused by numerous metals commonly used in costume jewelry. The most common of these are nickel, chrome, and mercury. Many types of costume jewelry, as well as wristwatches, zippers, snaps, and hooks on clothing, contain nickel. Another source of the metals that cause allergic contact dermatitis is certain contact lens solutions containing mercury. If you are allergic to any of the metals commonly associated with allergic contact dermatitis, you should avoid products that contain mercury. Check the label of contact lens solutions; products are available that do not contain mercury. Avoid costume jewelry containing nickel, opting instead for stainless steel products or jewelry made from 14-karat gold. Even though gold also contains some nickel for strength, the nickel is bound by the gold and therefore usually doesn't cause a reaction.

Cosmetics, ranging from nail polish to hair dyes, are another source of allergens causing allergic contact dermatitis. Perhaps the most frequent offender is the chemical paraphenylenediamine, contained in some hair dyes. Again, if certain cosmetics or dyes cause you to have allergy attacks, the best solution is avoidance. There are hypoallergenic formulas available for most cosmetics, which are free of the dyes and chemicals implicated in causing many cases of allergic contact dermatitis. It is important to note, however, that "hypoallergenic formulation" does not mean without allergy. Therefore some people with allergies may have a reaction to certain hypoallergenic formulations. Even some medication creams can cause this skin allergy. Neomycin is the most offending agent and can be found in many antibiotic creams. Some steroid creams can also cause contact allergy. You should check with your doctor for products that do not contain allergy-causing chemicals.

Avoiding the substances that cause allergic contact dermatitis is the best therapy. But if you should come into contact with an allergy-causing substance, there are some things you can do.

Treating Allergic Contact Dermatitis

1. Wash clothing and other objects that have come into contact with a plant resin to avoid reexposure.

2. Antihistamine pills can usually stop the itching associated with this condition.

3. Try not to scratch. The rash from allergic contact dermatitis generally does not leave a scar unless excessive scratching causes an infection. The fluid from the rash does not spread the rash, but if

your hands are contaminated by the plant resin, scratching can spread the chemical.

4. Soothe the area with cold, wet compresses made from a solution of 2 ounces of vinegar in 1 gallon of water. Calamine lotion can also help ease the itching.

5. Steroid creams are perhaps the most effective treatment. You can buy nonprescription cortisone creams for mild reactions or ask your doctor for a stronger prescription cream or oral steroid if the reaction is severe. Excessive scratching may result in secondary infections, which may require antibiotics.

Insect Allergies

Allergic reactions to insect stings are a major medical problem. While the overwhelming majority of people are not allergic to insect stings, those who are can suffer serious allergic reactions. About 50 to 100 people die each year from allergic reactions to insect stings. These deaths are the result of anaphylactic reactions to the venom in the insect stings. It is important to remember that although you may be allergic to the venom of certain insects, you won't necessarily have an anaphylactic reaction if you are stung. However, if you are allergic to

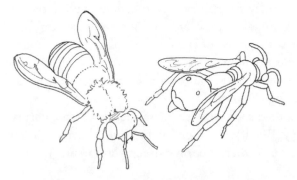

*The venom from bees and wasps can lead to anaphylaxis
in some people with allergies.*

certain insect stings, you should ask your doctor for an epinephrine anaphylaxis kit and keep the kit with you at all times, especially when you are outside in the spring, summer, and fall.

The main insects whose stings may cause allergic reactions are fire ants, hornets, yellow jackets, wasps, and bees. While millions of Americans are stung by these insects each year, only a small percent are truly allergic. Almost anyone, whether allergic or not, will experience certain symptoms after being stung. The usual reaction to the stings of bees and their cousins tends to last only a few hours, causing redness, swelling, pain, and itching at the site of the sting. Fire ant stings can cause a hive at the site of the sting that tends to subside within about an hour. This hive usually is followed by a small blister that appears within about 4 hours. As many as 50 percent of people who are stung by fire ants encounter swelling, itching, redness, and pain that can last for several days.

Among people who are truly allergic to the stings of fire ants and bees and their cousins, the venom can cause mast cells throughout the body to release histamine, leading to a possible anaphylactic reaction. The initial reaction can progress to include all the symptoms of an ana-phylactic reaction, as well as itching and hives over large areas of the body. This type of reaction should be taken seriously and treated immediately. If you are sensitive to the stings of any of these insects and you are stung, you should administer your epinephrine immediately and go to the nearest emergency room. Anaphylactic reactions to stinging insects are most common in allergic people who already have been sensitized to the insect venom from a previous sting.

"Rachel"

Rachel was three years old the first time she was stung by a bee. Although the event was traumatic, with the youngster crying and a small red welt appearing on her arm, her mother, Sally, did not think it was cause for alarm. She removed the stinger, wiped the area with some alcohol, and sent Rachel to play indoors for a while. By morning the swelling had eased and Rachel had almost forgotten about the incident.

It was not for another 10 years that Rachel was stung again. The reaction that time was quite different. The family was on a camping trip, and while hiking Rachel was stung on her arm. Mom had a first-aid kit in her backpack, so the family stopped while Dad removed the stinger. But shortly afterward, Rachel began feeling ill. She complained of a headache and began to feel sick to her stomach, and her entire arm where the bee had stung her began to swell. The family cut short their hike and headed back for camp, worried but confident that Rachel's only problem was that she had exerted herself too much. Sally, Rachel's mother, recalls thinking that her daughter's symptoms probably were not related to the bee sting. "I remembered that when she was stung before, nothing had happened, so we really weren't too concerned about the sting," she says.

By the time they got back to their tent, however, Rachel's condition was worsening. The family piled into the car and drove to the nearest hospital, which fortunately was only about 20 minutes away. When they arrived, Rachel was even worse. She was very tired, hives had begun to break out on her body, she was having trouble breathing, and she was feeling dizzy. Doctors in the emergency room quickly gave her an injection of epinephrine. After about 20 minutes Rachel seemed to be doing better, and the doctors administered a second injection. Soon after, Rachel was exhausted from the experience but no worse for wear.

Back home, Sally took Rachel to the family doctor and explained what had happened on their camping trip. The doctor said it was likely that Rachel had had an anaphylactic reaction and that she was extremely allergic to bee stings. "I had heard of anaphylaxis, but I wasn't really sure what it meant and I certainly didn't think Rachel had it," Sally says. She told the doctor that this was not the first time Rachel had been stung by a bee and that the first time the reaction seemed normal. "But he explained that some people who are prone to anaphylaxis do not react so forcefully the first few times they are stung; that the first stings cause the body to remember the toxin in the bee sting, so that it causes a much bigger reaction in the future," she says.

The doctor told Sally and Rachel that anaphylaxis is a serious allergic reaction that if not treated immediately can cause coma and death. He prescribed an anaphylaxis emergency kit and told Rachel to keep it on her at all times. He then taught Sally and Rachel how to administer the epinephrine injection in the kit and how to take the pills about 20 minutes after the shot. "It was scary to know that my daughter could actually die from a bee sting, but now we know more about anaphylaxis and how to treat it," Sally says. "It hasn't stopped us from hiking and taking family camping trips, but we are sure to always have a kit on hand."

Rachel is 20 years old now, and she is never without her anaphylaxis kit. "I keep one in my purse and one in my car so I'll always have it available," Rachel says. "It doesn't interfere with my life; it's something you learn to live with. Of course, I am a little nervous around bees." ❏

While anaphylaxis is the most serious allergic reaction to stinging insects, local reactions can pose significant discomfort. If you are stung by one of these insects and do not develop the signs of an anaphylactic reaction, there are some things you can do to ease the pain, itching, and swelling.

Treating Localized Insect Stings

1. Elevate the part of the body stung and apply ice or a cold compress to reduce the swelling. Do not break any blister that may form.

2. Clean the blisters with soap and water to prevent an infection.

3. Topical steroid creams and oral antihistamines can help relieve the itching from these stings.

4. Severe stings may require oral steroids to reduce the swelling. If you have a severe sting, see your doctor.

5. Seek immediate medical attention if the swelling progresses.

Allergy shots using tiny and increasing doses of the venom are an effective way to desensitize someone who has had systemic allergic reactions to stinging insects. These shots work in the same way as allergy shots for ragweed, discussed in detail in chapter 8. If you are allergic to stinging insects, ask your doctor if venom immunotherapy can help. As with all allergies, avoidance is the best therapy for allergies to stinging insects. You can reduce your chance of being stung by wearing closed-toed shoes, socks, gloves, and insect repellent when gardening, and identifying and exterminating hives and ant mounds near your home.

Latex Allergy

Allergy to latex has been increasing rapidly for the last 15 years. Doctors believe that the increase in the number of people allergic to latex is caused by greater use of the substance in everyday products. A milky-white substance derived from the rubber tree, latex is found in products ranging from medical equipment to toys to household goods to condoms. These products can cause allergic reactions ranging from skin rashes to anaphylaxis. In fact, allergy to latex has been blamed for a number of fatal and severe anaphylactic reactions. However, there are a number of products labeled as latex that actually contain no trace of the substance. Latex paint, for example, contains no latex or rubber products. While some people complain of eye itchiness, nasal congestion, or difficulty breathing when exposed to the fumes of latex paint, this is not a true latex allergy.

Those at the greatest risk of developing an allergy to latex appear to be homemakers and health care workers, who have repeated exposure to latex gloves, and children with medical conditions such as spina bifida, which requires multiple surgeries. These conditions and surgeries increase the children's exposure to latex medical devices.

Latex allergy occurs in the same manner as most other allergies; that is, it is a response by IgE antibodies to a substance viewed as harmful to the body. The allergy tends to develop after repeated exposure to latex, in much the same way as other allergies that require the body's immune system to develop a memory of the substance so it can react when reexposed in the future. While it is still difficult to predict if someone is allergic to latex, doctors have found that the condition is more common among people with family members who have other allergies. Recently doctors have found that people allergic to bananas, avocados, and chestnuts are most at risk of developing an allergy to latex. Those allergic to certain fruits and vegetables, including apples, carrots, celery, papaya, kiwi, potato, tomato, and melon, may also be at risk of developing latex allergy, although the association between these allergies is not so clearly understood.

SOME COMMON PRODUCTS THAT CONTAIN LATEX

Adhesive bandages

Adhesive cement

Baby bottle nipples

Balloons

Bathing caps

Blood pressure cuffs and tubing

Cervical caps and dilators

Condoms

Cosmetic sponges

Diaphragms

Door and window insulation

Elastic bands and threads sewn into clothing

Erasers

Household and surgical gloves

Hot-water bottles

Pacifiers

Plungers

Rubber hand grips on racquets, bicycles, garden tools, and other products

Rubber clothing, such as raincoats

Rubber toys and balls

Shoes

Shower curtains

Spandex

If you are allergic to latex, your symptoms may range from mild to severe depending on the type of product to which you are exposed and the severity of your allergies. Avoiding products that contain latex is the best way to manage this allergy. If you suspect that you or a family member is allergic to latex, see your doctor immediately. He or she may prescribe an anaphylaxis kit—described earlier in this chapter—if it appears that your allergy has the potential to become severe.

Food Allergies

Food allergies are among the most controversial and most difficult to diagnose of all allergies. Though the observation that certain foods can cause allergic reactions dates to the ancient Greek physician Hippocrates, who first noted that cow's milk could cause health problems in some people, there still are no clear estimates of the number of people affected by food allergies. Part of the problem is the wide range of reactions that can stem from ingesting certain foods, thus leading to difficulties in defining what a food allergy really is. Further muddying the field of food allergies has been the rise to prominence of certain offshoots of the field of allergy. These disciplines hold that a wide array of substances can lead to very minor, undefined symptoms in people who may be mildly sensitive. Unlike the field of allergy, which relies on well-respected tests to document an allergy to a certain substance, these less traditional branches of medicine believe that a person's reaction to certain substances may be so mild that it does not show up on traditional tests, yet still can cause symptoms. (These unproven avenues of allergy and asthma research are discussed in chapter 11.)

Foods can cause a number of reactions, not all of which are true allergies. Some possible reactions to foods include the following:

Food intolerance is an abnormal reaction to a food or food additive. Unlike a true allergy, it has no proven immunologic basis. For example, some people may be intolerant to milk sugar, or lactose, because they lack the enzyme needed to properly digest the substance.

Food poisoning is a reaction to toxins, bacteria, or other parasites in contaminated foods.

Pharmacologic food reaction is a known adverse effect to a food additive or naturally occurring chemical in a food. For example, some people develop nervous jitters from the caffeine in coffee.

Food allergy is an allergic reaction to a food or food additive that is orchestrated by the same IgE and mast cell reactions responsible for hay fever and other allergies. This type of reaction can lead to nausea, vomiting, diarrhea, hives, swelling of lips, eyes, and tongue, and possibly anaphylaxis.

About 6 percent of children under age 2 have true food allergies, although the majority of these reactions fade by the tenth birthday, with between 1 and 2 percent of children over age 10 truly allergic to certain foods. The most common food allergens are cow's milk, eggs, peanuts, certain shellfish, and nuts. Since peanuts are a legume and not a true nut, you may be allergic to peanuts but not to cashews or other nuts. However, it is possible to be allergic to both peanuts and nuts. Food allergies are a possible source of anaphylaxis, the potentially fatal reaction discussed earlier in this chapter. Foods most commonly associated with anaphylaxis are peanuts, nuts, shellfish, eggs, and seeds such as sesame.

The most common type of allergic reaction that occurs as the result of eating certain foods is hives: red, itchy, swollen areas that appear suddenly on the skin and last about 24 hours or less. Since foods are digested in the stomach and intestines, other reactions may include vomiting, diarrhea, and abdominal cramping. Food allergies have also been linked to a red rash around the mouth, itching and swelling of the mouth, and a scratchy feeling in the throat. Some studies also indicate that food allergies can trigger asthma attacks in people with asthma. About 8 percent of children with asthma may experience breathing problems that are triggered by food allergies. Because not all children with asthma also have food allergies, the allergies alone are responsible for triggering asthma in less than 10 percent of children with asthma.

A study published by the American Lung Association found that the foods most commonly linked to triggering asthma attacks are milk, eggs, and soy or wheat products. The study looked at 26 children with asthma who were allergic to eggs, wheat, milk, soy, or fish. Researchers hid dehydrated versions of the allergy-provoking foods in capsules and administered the capsules to the children. They found that 12 of the children experienced asthma symptoms, including coughing, wheezing, itchy throat, and chest tightness. Of the 12 children with food allergy–provoked asthma symptoms, 7 had signs of airway inflammation, the early sign of an impending asthma attack. Other studies of children at risk for anaphylactic reactions from certain foods found that children with asthma are at greater risk for severe food allergic reactions than children without asthma.

Food allergies are diagnosed in much the same manner as other allergies. The physician takes a careful history of the patient's symptoms and administers the skin or RAST tests described in chapter 7. These tests determine which foods may possibly trigger an allergic reaction. Foods that cause a positive reaction on the tests are then removed from the diet for a few weeks. Then food challenges, in which the person with allergies tries small amounts of the suspect foods, can be performed at home to determine the offending substances.

Armed with this knowledge, the best offense against food allergies is a good defense: weeding these foods from the diet and carefully avoiding foods that may contain minute traces of allergens. People with food allergies must be especially careful when dining out and must check all the ingredients on packaged foods. Traces of foods that can cause allergies may be contained in food products that otherwise pose no danger. For instance, crushed nuts can be an ingredient in salad dressings; oils from seeds and nuts may be used during food preparation; and peanuts may be used as a garnish or dressing. Traces of peanuts can even be found in some plain chocolate candies. If a person with a food allergy accidentally eats a food that triggers an allergic reaction, an epinephrine injection contained in one of the anaphylaxis kits described earlier in this chapter is the first treatment. The antihistamine diphenhydramine, found in the drug Benadryl, is helpful with minor reactions such as small hives.

DID YOU KNOW...?

In trying to build a better soybean, genetic engineers found that it's possible to transfer an allergen from one food to another.

While attempting to boost the nutritional properties of soybeans by adding genes from the nutrient-heavy Brazil nut, the genetic researchers found that they also transferred the nut's allergic material to the tiny soybean. That means that people with an allergy to Brazil nuts but not to soybeans could have an allergic reaction if they were to eat the new soybean.

The company that was trying to make the hardier soybean stopped its research after it discovered that it had turned the soybean into a possible allergen. No one ate the newfangled soybean before the researchers discontinued the project. The news raised concern that unsuspecting people with other allergies may inadvertently expose themselves to allergens in genetically altered foods that previously caused no reactions.

With an increasing number of companies turning to genetic engineering to rev up the nutritional and growing abilities of some plant foods, this nutty soybean shows that researchers and people with allergies alike will have to be increasingly vigilant to old foods that may be genetically altered.

Can Allergies Be Prevented in Children?

Developing allergies is a two-part process: first, children must inherit the gene or genes that leave them at risk; second, they must be repeatedly exposed to an allergen so their immune system develops a memory of the substance via the allergy antibody IgE. While you can't control what genes your children inherit, you can reduce the chance that they will develop allergies by following some guidelines. These guidelines are designed to reduce your child's exposure to substances that are known allergens. While children cannot avoid exposure to allergens throughout their lives, some research indicates that exposure early in life may be the most important when it comes to fostering immune system memory.

To begin with, pregnant women should maintain a well-balanced diet and avoid bingeing on any one food. After birth, breastfeeding for four to six months may reduce the chance that your child will develop allergies. While breastfeeding, you should avoid giving your newborn any solid foods for about the first six months of life. You can supplement your child's diet with a milk- or soy-based formula prior to weaning. While doctors still do not know whether avoiding certain foods within the first six months of life is protective against allergies, it appears that the fewer the number of foods introduced during this time, the better. When you do begin to introduce new foods into your child's diet, you should start slowly, gradually adding a small amount on the first day and increasing the amount over the next four to seven days. Be sure to watch for signs of possible allergies, such as a rash, stomach upset, coughing, or respiratory problems. If you see these signs, discontinue the food and contact your doctor. The signs may indicate an allergy, or they may merely be coincidental to the development of some viral infection or stomach illness. It is best to add no more than one new food to your child's diet every four to seven days.

One possible plan for introducing foods to the diets of children whose parents have allergies is as follows:

• At 7 months, begin with small amounts of vegetables and rice.

• At 8 months, increase the amount of rice and rice cereals.

• At 9 months, try introducing small amounts of meat, but avoid fish.

• At 10 months, begin giving your child noncitrus fruit.

After your child's first birthday you can begin introducing other grains, legumes, corn, and citrus fruits to the diet. When adding new foods to your child's diet, you should avoid some highly allergenic foods, perhaps for as long as the first two years of life. These foods include eggs, peanuts, chocolate, fish, strawberries, and nuts.

You should also try to minimize your child's exposure to other allergens and irritants. First and most important is not to smoke. Studies published by the American Lung Association have found that the children of parents who smoke are three to four times more likely to develop asthma than children of nonsmoking parents. Of course, there are many other reasons to stop smoking, including reducing your risk of lung cancer, emphysema, chronic bronchitis, heart disease, and stroke.

Next, you should try to keep animals out of the home and away from the child. Your baby-sitter's home should also be free of pets. Exposure to furry and feathered pets can sensitize children with a predisposition to allergies. If you or your spouse has allergies or asthma, reduce your child's exposure to mold spores and dust mites by keeping his or her bedroom as clean as possible, washing bedding in hot water, and using allergy-free cases for mattresses and pillows. Even though the bed is covered with linens, it will not be protected from house dust mites because of the air holes in the sides of the mattress. Avoid carpeting in the child's bedroom because it is a haven for dust mites and mold spores. Try also to keep children away from freshly mowed lawns, raked leaves, and other sources of pollen.

10 / Asthma and Pregnancy

WHEN YOU ARE PREGNANT, YOU ARE BREATHING FOR TWO, and that can be especially hard for women who have asthma. Asthma is one of the most common diseases that complicate pregnancy, affecting about 4 percent of all pregnancies. The effects of asthma in pregnancy can be profound, ranging from premature birth to maternal and fetal death. But asthma in pregnancy can be controlled. Women with asthma should not fear getting pregnant or giving birth; it is simply a matter of properly monitoring the disease and getting the proper asthma medications.

Because asthma attacks can occur faster and be more severe in pregnant women, doctors recommend that they have regular lung function and peak expiratory flow tests. Pregnant women with asthma should monitor their peak flow at least twice a day. The regular ultrasound you will get during the twelfth to twentieth week of your pregnancy is probably enough to monitor your fetus. If you have severe asthma, your doctor may recommend additional ultrasounds to be performed during the second and third trimesters of pregnancy.

If you have an asthma attack during labor, your obstetrician will want to monitor your heart rate and peak flow rates during the remaining labor. Continuous electronic fetal heart monitoring during labor may be necessary for women with severe asthma.

Controlling your exposure to asthma triggers is of primary importance during pregnancy. (See chapter 6 for more about measures to trigger-proof your home.) Special preventive measures in pregnancy include a flu shot to prevent a bout of the flu. (Later in this chapter we'll discuss whether you should get a flu shot during pregnancy and, if so, when during your pregnancy you should get it.) A flu shot can significantly reduce your risk of certain respiratory infections, which are potent asthma triggers in pregnancy. While there is no way to avoid getting the common cold, which also can trigger your asthma, following some commonsense advice may help. Avoid contact with people who have a cold, and wash your hands as much as possible if you are with someone who has the sniffles. And follow your mother's warnings: avoid a draft and don't go out in the rain without your umbrella.

The best asthma control in pregnancy results when there is a partnership between the patient, the physician treating her asthma, and the obstetrician. When you become pregnant, you should make sure that your obstetrician has all the information necessary to control your asthma while making sure your pregnancy proceeds normally. If possible, you should pick an obstetrician who is familiar with asthma and who has treated other pregnant women with asthma. You should also have the physician treating your asthma update your obstetrician on your disease. To make the most of your first visit with your obstetrician, you should bring along a complete history of your asthma, including what medications you take and how often you take them. Use the Asthma History Checklist for Pregnant Women, on the next page, as a guideline.

The risks to the mother or fetus from uncontrolled asthma are far greater than the risks from the medications used to control asthma. It is important for pregnant women to have their asthma under good control: breathing difficulties affect the fetus by compromising the oxygen supply. When asthma is controlled, women with asthma have no more complications during pregnancy and labor than other women. However, uncontrolled asthma during pregnancy can produce serious maternal and fetal complications.

A study published by the American Lung Association supports the idea that it is riskier to leave a woman's asthma uncontrolled than to use asthma medication during pregnancy. Doctors studied more than 800 pregnant women, about half of whom had asthma. The women with asthma kept a regular asthma diary of their symptoms and medications and were evaluated by an asthma specialist once a month. Although the women with asthma all received medications to control their breathing and reduce their chance of an attack, the researchers found no difference in the rates of infant deaths, birth defects, preterm births, low-birth-weight infants, or growth retardation between the women with asthma and those without. The study supported the hypothesis that most asthma medications are safe during pregnancy.

On the other hand, uncontrolled asthma during pregnancy can

result in a host of complications to both the expectant mother and the fetus. Uncontrolled asthma is associated with complications such as:

- premature birth
- low birth weight
- maternal blood pressure changes (a serious condition known as preeclampsia)

ASTHMA HISTORY CHECKLIST FOR PREGNANT WOMEN

1. I first was diagnosed with asthma _____ years ago.
2. I experience attacks of wheezing _____ times a week.
3. I have trouble breathing at night _____ times a month.
4. I have trouble breathing when exposed to:
   (List the asthma promoters and triggers that cause you to have an asthma attack. See chapter 3 for a detailed description of common asthma promoters and triggers.)

   _____

   _____

   _____

   _____

   _____

5. I am currently taking the following drugs to control my breathing:
   (List the asthma drugs you are taking and how often you take them.)

   _____

   _____

   _____

   _____

6. I measure my peak expiratory flow rates _____ times a day, at _____ o'clock and _____ o'clock.
7. My best peak expiratory flow rate is _____.

In general, about one-third of women with asthma notice more trouble breathing during pregnancy; another one-third find that their asthma is actually under better control during pregnancy; and the last one-third notice no changes in their asthma. Asthma is under good control if the expectant mother is:

- Active without experiencing any asthma symptoms

- Sleeping through the night and not waking because of asthma symptoms

- Attaining her personal best peak flow number. (This is an important indicator of asthma in pregnancy, as it is the most objective way you can measure your own lung function.)

Controlling Asthma During Pregnancy

It is of utmost importance that pregnant women with asthma strive to achieve the best possible control of their symptoms. If you are pregnant, you should try to reduce your chance of having an asthma attack by:

- Controlling your environment and reducing your exposure to asthma triggers.

- Continuing regularly scheduled medications during pregnancy and labor and delivery.

- Getting an influenza vaccine after the first three months of pregnancy. The flu vaccine is recommended for women with identified viral infections as one of their asthma triggers.

- Exercising moderately. Many people with asthma suffer an attack following vigorous exercise. Pregnant women with asthma should exercise under the supervision of their physician. Exercise-induced asthma attacks can be avoided or reduced by taking medication before exercise, including a warm-up and cool-down as part of the exercise, and wearing a scarf over the mouth and nose if exercising in very cold air. (Exercise-induced asthma is discussed in detail in chapter 15.)

- Avoiding tobacco smoke. The fetus can be exposed to the chemicals in environmental tobacco smoke (secondhand smoke) from either the mother or father. This exposure may have adverse effects. Studies have found that infants are three times more likely to die of Sudden Infant Death Syndrome (SIDS) if their mothers smoked during or after pregnancy. Secondhand tobacco smoke is a potent asthma trigger that you should avoid to reduce your chance of an attack. A pregnant woman who smokes runs a greatly increased risk of having a severe asthma episode at some time in the pregnancy, which can in turn result in a low-birth-weight baby.

Monitoring Asthma During Pregnancy

Regular measurements of your lung function should be performed throughout your pregnancy. These tests are essential for assessing and monitoring whether your asthma is under control, so you and your doctor can make appropriate changes to your medications. If you are pregnant, your doctor should perform tests of your lung function at every obstetrical visit. These tests should include an office spirometry and peak expiratory flow rate test. You can also perform peak flow testing at home. Ideally, your lung function should change little during pregnancy. (See chapter 5 for more information on peak flow testing.)

While you are pregnant, many of the routine tests performed by your obstetrician can help determine if your asthma is affecting the growth of your fetus. The routine ultrasound scans you receive throughout pregnancy can provide an early indication of how your fetus is growing; slow or reduced growth may indicate that your fetus is not getting enough oxygen, and one reason for that may be your asthma. During this test a gel is put on the abdomen, and a hand-held sensor provides an image of the fetus that is projected onto a computer screen. An electronic fetal heart rate monitor may also be used to assure fetal well-being.

Asthma During Labor and Delivery

Your due date is now near, and your bag is packed for the trip to the hospital. You have successfully managed your asthma throughout your pregnancy, and it is finally time to give birth. But your asthma management does not stop here.

The mother and fetus are both monitored during labor and delivery to ensure the good health of both. This is especially necessary for women with asthma. The fetus is usually monitored electronically upon your admission to the hospital. If your asthma is under control, continuous monitoring may not be necessary. If your doctor finds that your asthma is acting up, however, or if you are at high risk for an attack during pregnancy, the doctor may consider continuous fetal monitoring throughout delivery.

You should expect to have a peak flow rate taken on admission for labor and delivery and every 12 hours following. If asthma symptoms develop, peak flow rates should be measured again after you receive asthma treatments. Don't be afraid to ask for adequate pain relief during delivery, as reducing pain may lower the risk of an asthma attack.

Asthma and the Postnatal Period

Your beautiful new addition to the family has arrived. What can you expect next?

After the baby is born, it may be necessary to change your asthma medications and doses. Because some women experience changes in their asthma during pregnancy, the asthma may change again following delivery. Because the postnatal period can involve anxiety about the newborn, fatigue, and possibly significant postpartum depression, you must be extra vigilant about controlling your asthma.

You should also rest assured that most of the commonly used asthma medications are safe to use while breastfeeding. Inhaled bronchodilators and inhaled anti-inflammatories do not appear to cause side effects in breastfed newborns whose mothers have asthma. However, there are some exceptions. Theophylline has been found to make its way into breast milk and can make your baby irritable. Antihistamines should be avoided because they can cause sleeplessness and irritability in children.

COMMONLY ASKED QUESTIONS ABOUT ASTHMA IN PREGNANCY

Can asthma affect my pregnancy?

Studies indicate that most women with asthma have normal pregnancies and that the disease, when properly controlled, does not increase the risk of maternal or fetal complications. Poorly controlled asthma, however, can result in dangers to the expectant mother and pregnancy complications such as low birth weight and premature birth.

Why does uncontrolled asthma affect my pregnancy?

When asthma is out of control, pregnant women do not get enough oxygen. The decrease in oxygen in the expectant mother's blood may lead to a drop in the amount of oxygen reaching the fetus. This lack of oxygen can impair fetal growth and development.

Can my asthma medications hurt my fetus?

Most asthma medications appear to be safe when used during pregnancy, and the risk of uncontrolled asthma to the fetus far outweighs any risk from the medications. Inhaled beclomethasone (a steroid), anti-inflammatories, and beta-adrenergic drugs have all received a clean bill of health when used in pregnancy. Oral steroids and theophylline may pose more of a risk and are reserved for pregnant women with severe asthma or those experiencing a severe attack. Remember, however, that poorly controlled asthma in the mother is more dangerous to the baby than any of these drugs.

Does asthma worsen during pregnancy?

About one-third of pregnant women with asthma find their breathing gets worse during pregnancy; another one-third experience no change in their asthma; and the remaining third find that their asthma symptoms actually get better during pregnancy.

When during pregnancy is my asthma most likely to change?

If your asthma is going to worsen during pregnancy, it appears it is most likely to do so during the late second and early third trimesters. Asthma attacks late in pregnancy and during labor and delivery are very rare.

Can I use Lamaze if I have asthma?

Yes, most women with asthma are able to perform Lamaze breathing techniques.

Can I breastfeed if I use my asthma medications?

Women with asthma should be encouraged to breastfeed. The most commonly used asthma medications, such as inhaled steroids, anti-inflammatories like cromolyn, and inhaled beta-adrenergic drugs do not appear to be taken up by breast milk. Traces of oral steroids, theophylline, and some oral antihistamines have been found in breast milk and may have effects on the newborn. You should ask your doctor about the asthma drugs you are using and whether they are safe to be used when you are breastfeeding.

Asthma Medications During Pregnancy

While most commonly used asthma medications are safe in pregnancy, pregnant women with asthma may need special doses of these drugs. Doctors working for the federal government's National Asthma Education and Prevention Program's Working Group on Asthma and

Pregnancy have developed recommended doses of asthma drugs in pregnancy. Here is a summary of their recommendations.

Inhaled adrenergic drugs: Any inhaled adrenergic drug is safe during pregnancy. Pregnant women with mild chronic asthma should use 2 puffs when they are wheezing and before exposure to exercise or allergens. Women with chronic moderate or chronic severe asthma can take up to 2 puffs every 4 hours.

Inhaled cromolyn or nedocromil: These drugs are safe during pregnancy and can reduce airway inflammation and the chance of allergen- or exercise-induced asthma attacks. Pregnant women with mild chronic asthma should use 2 puffs before exposure to exercise or allergens. Women with chronic moderate or chronic severe asthma can take up to 2 puffs 4 times a day to reduce the inflammation in their airways.

Inhaled steroids: Doctors recommend the drug beclomethasone for use in pregnancy. Pregnant women with chronic moderate or chronic severe asthma should take 2 to 5 puffs 2 to 4 times a day to reduce their airway inflammation.

Oral steroids: If oral steroids are needed to control asthma during pregnancy, doctors recommend using the drug prednisone. This drug should be used only by women with chronic severe asthma who are not getting adequate control of their symptoms from other asthma medications. Pregnant women should take burst courses of 40 mg a day in 1 or 2 doses for one week and then taper off the drug for one week. If you need a longer course of oral steroids to control your asthma in pregnancy, doctors recommend a single morning dose taken every other day to minimize side effects.

If you are pregnant or are considering getting pregnant, having asthma should not be a deterrent. Pregnant women can monitor and control their disease just like anyone else with asthma. Women with properly controlled asthma should have no problems carrying a child and giving birth. The key is planning. Once you find that you are pregnant, tell your obstetrician that you have asthma. If your obstetrician is not familiar with controlling asthma, tell him or her about the National Asthma Education and Prevention Program's Executive Summary on the Management of Asthma During Pregnancy. Your doctor can get this document from the federal government's National Heart, Lung, and Blood Institute. You can aid your obstetrician in managing your asthma during pregnancy by bringing him or her a list of the asthma medications you are using, how often you use them, and a description of your breathing problems. Use the checklist on page 136 as a guide in preparing this information. If you have an asthma management plan based on your peak expiratory flow rates that you developed with your asthma specialist, you also should show that plan to your obstetrician.

11 / Controversial Theories and Therapies

IT IS A PARADOX THAT AS THE UNDERSTANDING OF ASTHMA AND allergies has increased, fields that advance unproven approaches to testing and treating these conditions have flourished. To be sure, there is still much that mainstream medicine does not understand about these twin conditions, yet what is known about diagnosing and treating them has exploded in recent years.

The approaches to diagnosing and treating asthma and allergies presented in this book are based on accepted medical practice generally backed up by solid clinical studies. But there are many health practitioners who rely on unconventional or unproven methods that generally have no scientific basis. They may be age-old folk remedies revived and revised for a modern audience, or they may be theories developed in reaction to many of the ills of modern-day life, such as pollution. Whatever the approach, these unproven therapies, which are likely to be ineffective, can be quite appealing to some people.

A diagnosis of allergies or asthma based on an unproven set of tests may comfort people who suffer from a diffuse set of symptoms such as malaise, fatigue, and headaches. Unproven tests that purport to show a diagnosis of asthma or allergies may seem like an answer to people who have been to traditional doctors but have found little relief from their conditions. Unless the tests and therapies have proven effectiveness, however, these people may be throwing away their money and endangering themselves. Many conditions have symptoms that mimic those of allergies and asthma—headaches, fatigue, sneezing, itchy eyes, and wheezing. People who get an incorrect diagnosis of these conditions when another disease is actually the cause of their complaints can be delaying much-needed therapy while waiting for an unproven or inappropriate treatment to work. A host of other diseases can cause these symptoms.

Remember that the way to live a healthy life with allergies and asthma is to manage them properly. This can start only with a proper diagnosis and a treatment plan that includes medications to reverse and prevent some attacks. Also, among the best therapies for allergies and asthma is avoidance of the triggers that can cause an attack. The best way to start managing your disease properly is by seeing a specialist who can recognize your condition, conduct the tests needed to determine what triggers your disease, and prescribe a treatment plan. (More information about the different types of doctors you should see is given in chapter 12.)

Clinical Ecology

If your problem is not readily diagnosed by your primary-care physician, it is important to go to medical doctors specializing in allergy or asthma rather than physicians and other health care providers operating on the fringe of what is currently known as acceptable medicine. Among the most highly publicized of these practitioners is a group of doctors known as clinical ecologists. Clinical ecology relates to a theory held by some doctors that people can suffer from a wide range of symptoms after repeated and prolonged exposure to common substances in the environment. Clinical ecologists believe that sensitivities to a variety of chemicals and food additives can confuse the immune system so it can no longer distinguish between nutritious foods and toxic chemicals. The result, they believe, is an overproduction of antibodies to normal foods, leading the body to react with a host of symptoms. These symptoms and diseases include:

- behavioral disorders
- depression
- chronic fatigue
- schizophrenia
- learning disabilities
- arthritis
- gastrointestinal problems
- respiratory problems
- urinary complaints

The term *sensitivity* is often used by clinical ecologists because the reaction to these substances does not show up on any traditional allergy test. Clinical ecologists believe this is because the reaction is too small to trigger a traditionally used skin test.

Approaches to treating this so-called multiple chemical sensitivity syndrome include drastic diet alterations, such as eliminating all processed foods containing any trace of coloring or flavoring agents. Total elimination diets consisting solely of spring water followed by the gradual introduction of foods may be suggested. A clinical ecologist may also suggest that a person live and work only in spaces with filtered air and no synthetic materials. The final approach consists of treating people with diluted versions of the suspected allergens by injections or with drops placed under the tongue.

Currently there is little clear scientific evidence to support the approach to the above-mentioned problems; further studies are needed. A report by the American Lung Association and other groups concluded that a person who believes he or she suffers from multiple chemical sensitivity should receive a thorough medical workup to determine whether there is an underlying medical problem, and consultation with an allergist or other specialist may be warranted.

Unconventional Diagnostic Tests

A proper history and physical examination are the most important elements when making a diagnosis of asthma or allergies. Your doctor probably will follow up by having you undergo many of the asthma and allergy tests described earlier in this book. Among those are the tests of lung function to determine how efficiently your lungs are working and the skin tests to determine to which substances you are allergic. While any one of these tests alone cannot diagnose or predict allergies and asthma, taken together with a careful history of your symptoms, they can paint a clear picture of your condition.

In addition to these well-documented tests of allergy and asthma are tests used by some physicians and health practitioners that most reputable doctors believe have no value whatsoever. You should know a little about these tests so that you can distinguish them from accepted medical tests in your search for a proper treatment plan to control your asthma and allergies.

Cytotoxic Testing

Also known as the leukocytotoxic test or Bryan's test, this procedure is used by some physicians and laboratories who claim they can diagnose allergies to substances by mixing the suspected allergens in a test tube and adding a sample of the patient's white blood cells. The physician then looks at the blood cells under a microscope to check for any changes in shape or appearance. Proponents of cytotoxic testing say that swelling or other changes in the cells indicates that the person is allergic to whatever substance was in the test tube.

Numerous clinical trials conducted by research physicians have found that there is no difference in the reaction of white blood cells of people with or without allergies when exposed to allergens in test tubes. The test bears no relationship to the RAST and IgE skin tests discussed earlier in this book, which test for the presence of specific allergic responses or antibodies. Further, there is no proof that the test can diagnose food or other allergies. The test has been branded ineffective by the California State Court of Appeals, the Food and Drug Administration, and Medicare, which does not pay for the test because there is no evidence to support its use.

Provocation and Neutralization Technique

Proponents claim that this technique can diagnose allergies to foods, inhaled substances, environmental chemicals, hormones, and certain fungi. It is performed by exposing a person to the suspected allergen either by injection or by a drop placed under the tongue. The patient is then asked to record any sensation or symptom he or she experiences during the following 10 minutes. The appearance of any type of feeling or symptom is interpreted as a positive result, meaning the person is allergic to that substance. If the test is negative, it is repeated with increasingly higher doses until the patient reports feeling something. The patient is then given a lower concentration of the substance, and if fewer or no symptoms are reported, the reaction is said to be neutralized. This neutralizing dose is then used as a therapy for the condition, a process discussed later in this chapter.

There is no basis for the use of this test. The understanding of the immune system negates the possibility that symptoms can be immediately neutralized under the conditions used in this test. Numerous trials have been conducted to determine the validity of this test, most of which have failed to show it can diagnose allergies. For example, a study of 18 people undergoing the test to diagnose food allergies found no difference in their reports of symptoms whether a food extract or placebo drop was used.

A variation of the test used to diagnose breathing problems is similarly fraught with problems. This test, conducted in testing booths called Environmental Control Units, exposes people to airborne chemicals in an attempt to trigger and diagnose asthma symptoms. No controlled studies have been performed to check the test's effectiveness, and it should be noted that this form of testing bears no resemblance to the asthma tests discussed earlier in this book. However, reputable pulmonary laboratories do use a carefully controlled version of this test to diagnose asthma caused by occupationally encountered allergens.

Electrodermal Diagnosis

This test purports to measure changes in the electrical resistance of the skin when it is exposed to food allergens. The food extract is placed in a glass vial on an aluminum plate that is connected in the middle of an electrical circuit between the skin and a device used to measure electricity. If there is a decrease in skin resistance when a food allergen is placed in the circuit, a positive diagnosis is made. There is neither a rational basis for this test, nor have studies been performed to support its use.

Applied Kinesiology

In this test the muscle strength of a limb is measured before and after a food allergen, encased in a glass vial, is placed on the patient's skin. A technician subjectively measures the strength of the limb. If any weakness is judged to occur, the patient is considered to be allergic to the substance. Again, there is no rational basis for this test, nor is it plausible that an allergen can affect muscle strength or work its harm through a glass vial placed on the skin.

Unconventional Treatment Methods

The management plan for people with asthma or allergies is based on three forms of treatment: avoidance of allergens and asthma triggers, medications to reverse and prevent some attacks, and immunotherapy to desensitize people with allergies. All of the approaches to treatment discussed in this book have been developed under standard medical practice, and each has been evaluated in clinical studies to determine its effectiveness and safety. Unfortunately, there are a number of unproven, ineffective therapies being sold by people at the outskirts of traditional medicine.

Neutralization

Also known as symptom-relieving therapy, neutralization is an extension of the provocation and neutralization testing technique discussed above. Once that testing method purports to discover a suspected allergen, the person is given a liquid extract of the offending allergen. People are told to place a drop of the extract under their tongue when they anticipate being exposed to the substance in the environment. This method is also used for long-term maintenance therapy.

There is nothing to suggest that the immune system can respond to this type of therapy, especially when it comes to the immediate neutralization of an allergy. Neutralization treatment is usually prescribed for people with so-called chemical and food sensitivities rather than true allergies. Immunotherapy injections, discussed earlier in this book, work to lessen the sensitivity of people with allergies when given gradually over three to five years, which is not the same as giving the offending allergen only when needed before exposure. Very recent studies, however, indicate that carefully controlled immunization given orally may show promise for future immune therapies.

Urine Injections

Perhaps the most unconventional asthma and allergy treatment is based on the belief that injecting one's own sterilized urine back into the body can cure these conditions. This bizarre treatment holds that urine contains unspecified chemicals produced by the body during an allergic reaction and that these chemicals can inhibit or neutralize future allergy attacks. Although the drinking of urine is an ancient healing practice, there is no sound basis for this therapy. In fact, injecting urine can potentially be disastrous. Urine contains waste materials excreted by the body. Repeated injections of these waste materials can cause damage to the kidneys.

Unconventional Theories of Asthma and Allergies

Multiple Chemical Sensitivities

In the past 40 years, a group of physicians and other health practitioners has developed a theory that has gained a great deal of publicity through its use of catchy buzz words like "environmental illness," "20th-century disease," and "ecological sensitivity." The theory holds that a wide range of environmental chemicals can cause a variety of physical and psychological illnesses, from muscle and joint pain to gastrointestinal problems to fatigue and malaise. The overriding theory is that people suffer from these conditions because of failure of the human race to adapt to synthetic chemicals.

This theory is most often advocated by clinical ecologists who use the provocation and neutralization test techniques described earlier as a means of identifying people with multiple chemical sensitivities. Proponents may also use a variety of other tests in which they examine the blood and body tissues for signs of pesticides and other environmental chemicals. Treatment consists of the neutralization technique, megadoses of vitamins and mineral supplements, and avoidance of all offending chemicals, including exhaust fumes, scented household products, synthetic fabrics, plastics, and pesticides. Some people have gone so far as to establish "environmentally clean" communities in rural areas for people deemed unsuitable for the urban environment.

As with the other unconventional approaches to asthma and allergy discussed in this chapter, there is little scientific evidence regarding multiple chemical sensitivity. Diagnosing the condition is based on unproven testing methods, and none of the treatments have been evaluated by clinical studies.

Candidiasis Hypersensitivity Syndrome

Another school of allergy that exists on the fringe of medicine consists of practitioners who believe in something called the yeast sensitivity syndrome. This syndrome has been popularized in a number of books and holds that an overabundance of the yeast germ, *Candida albicans,* can cause a variety of symptoms, including fatigue, depression, hyperactivity, headache, skin problems, and breathing problems. Those who believe in the yeast syndrome purport that diets high in carbohydrates, and some medications such as antibiotics and birth control pills, can cause an overgrowth of the yeast germ in the body. This overgrowth, they believe, weakens the immune system, which is then more likely to react to foods, chemicals, and inhaled allergens.

The fact is that everyone has quantities of *Candida albicans* in their mouths and gastrointestinal tracts. The germ is not thought to cause any of the symptoms ascribed to it by believers in the yeast syndrome. Further, proponents of yeast hypersensitivity have diagnosed the condition in people who have never been exposed to birth control pills, antibiotics, or other factors thought to cause excessive growth of the germ. Diagnosis is made by a history only and is not confirmed by any type of testing. The recommended treatment consists of antifungal medications, vitamin and mineral supplements, and a diet devoid of sugar, yeast, and molds. There is no reason to believe in the yeast theory, and there are no studies hinting that it may be valid. And there is a risk that the long-term use of powerful antifungal drugs can cause dangerous, drug-resistant strains to grow in the body.

Protecting Yourself

If you think you have asthma or allergies, see a licensed medical practitioner. Remember that asthma and allergies are real conditions that can be accurately diagnosed by tests that have been evaluated in thousands of people. The proper diagnosis of asthma and allergies consists of a careful history and examination and the administration of proven tests to determine how severe your disease is and what allergens can trigger your attacks.

TESTS, TREATMENTS, AND THERAPIES TO AVOID

- Cytotoxic testing
- Provocation and neutralization technique
- Electrodermal diagnosis
- Applied kinesiology
- Neutralization
- Urine injections
- Clinical ecology
- Multiple chemical sensitivity
- Yeast syndrome

Once a diagnosis is made, you should develop an asthma or allergy maintenance plan with your doctor. Such a plan will allow you to take control of your disease and lead a normal life. You should be maintained on medications, proven to work in placebo-controlled clinical studies, that can reverse and even prevent some attacks. And you should employ the tips presented in chapter 6 on how to virtually trigger-proof your life. Numerous medically approved strategies for controlling asthma and allergies are explained in detail in earlier chapters, and you should follow them if you suspect that you or a family member has either of these conditions.

12 / The Family's Role

ASTHMA AND ALLERGIES ARE TRULY A FAMILY AFFAIR. CONTROL-ling asthma is an ongoing process, a way of living. It goes beyond simply taking medications. Proper control of asthma can be reached when all members of the family pull together as a team to help in the management and control of the person with asthma and allergies.

As we have seen, emotional stress can intensify or aggravate asthma attacks. By the very nature of asthma and allergies, children with these conditions live in a situation that makes for stress. First of all, there is fear—the fear during attacks of suffocation and the fear between episodes of their recurrence. Then there is the emotional blow that comes if the child is made to realize that he or she is somehow abnormal or different from other children—that he or she cannot study or play or live the way other children do. Such a blow can leave lifelong scars.

But the fact is that children with asthma are basically the same as other children. Children with asthma have the same high spirits, curiosity, alertness, and love of fun. Moreover, given recent advances in the way asthma is controlled and maintained, virtually all children with this disease can be pretty much like any other child, doing all the things children do. All it takes is the advice of a knowledgeable physician and some understanding and common sense on the part of family, teachers, playmates, and the children themselves.

The family's first duty is to find out as much as possible about asthma and about their child's specific condition. Families should encourage children with asthma to participate as much as possible in regular schoolwork, sports, and play, and help children explore new skills and interests. Apart from making the child with asthma feel capable, loved, and respected, the family's basic responsibility should be to help the child function in the same world in which other children live.

Parents should hesitate before placing a child in a special program. If the program is designed to help the child work and play alongside children without asthma, it can be worthwhile; or if it is designed to teach children how to control and live with their disease, it can be an excellent tool for children to gain independence. But if the program is based on the philosophy that children with asthma should be segregated from other children because they are different and have special needs, it may be of questionable value.

Teachers and school administrators should also encourage children with asthma to participate in the same classroom and recreational activities that other pupils take part in. But teachers should be aware of special problems that may occur among children with asthma. For instance, a child with asthma is more likely to be absent than is a healthy child and may seem drowsy or unable to concentrate as a result of necessary medications. Nevertheless, if teachers are informed, they know that a child with asthma is fully capable of doing just as well as anyone else—and they make sure that the child knows it too.

Of course, the other children may not be so understanding. They may not always accept a child who cannot participate in sports or play to the extent they do. If this is the case for your child, the other children need some instruction on asthma not only from teachers but from parents as well. With optimal therapy, more and more children with asthma are able to participate in competitive sports.

Teaching Children About Asthma

Parents should try to teach children with asthma about their condition, how to control it with medications, and what factors can trigger an attack. Well-educated children develop a sense of independence when they are able to manage their own disease. They become aware of what activities they can participate in and when they are likely to get into trouble with their asthma. And children are often the best teachers of other children. If your child knows how to manage and control his or her own disease and incorporates this management into his or her lifestyle, the chances are that other children will come to accept asthma and allergies as nothing out of the ordinary.

As children get older, they are able to take more responsibility for their daily activities, including management of their disease. The way this works best is when parents or adult helpers support the child as he or she takes on this increased responsibility. Try to let your child take on more responsibility as he or she gets older. Here are some helpful guidelines that you can use to help determine which responsibilities your child can take on at varying ages. Use the guidelines as a worksheet and check off the expectations that your child has completed. You can also have your child help track his or her own progress.

Preschoolers: Begin teaching preschoolers about their condition by getting them involved with their own asthma care.

- Teach them to cooperate with medicines and therapies.

- Train them in the correct techniques for taking medicines and other therapies.

- Give them their medications on a regular schedule so they develop the sense that asthma is best managed through a routine.

- Learn how the medications work and what side effects to watch for.

- Teach your child to recognize the symptoms of asthma.

- Teach your child to seek out help when he or she feels these symptoms.

- Begin using a peak flow meter and training your child in its proper use.

- Identify your child's asthma and allergy triggers, and control the amount of these triggers in your home.

School Age: Once children begin going to school, they are ready to take on more responsibility in controlling their own disease.

- Explain to school-age children what their medications do.

- Have them remind you when it is time for their regularly scheduled medications.

- Have them ask for any medications they may use before exercise.

- Continue to plan and oversee your child's routine medicines and therapies.

- Have them begin to monitor their own peak flow under your supervision.

- Let school-age children keep their own peak flow diary.

- Involve your child in treatment decisions based on peak flow readings, but retain the ultimate decision-making power.

- Explain the triggers that can make your child's asthma worse.

- Involve your child in identifying and controlling these triggers.

- Teach children that they should use their short-acting beta-adrenergic medications only to reverse attacks of wheezing.

Adolescents: By the time children reach their teens, they are mostly responsible for their own asthma management. But you can take this opportunity to fine-tune their program and educate them in some of the more complicated aspects of asthma care.

- Teens should be responsible for planning and taking their routine medicines and therapies.

- Take this opportunity to teach them about the side effects of their drugs and signs to watch for.

- Make sure they are always using the proper techniques when taking their medications or peak flow readings.

- Have them identify when their medications need to be refilled.

- Have teens talk with their doctor about their own treatment plan.

- Do spot checks of routine medicines and therapies.

- Have your child identify and know when to treat worsening asthma based on his or her peak flow readings.

- Explain to your teenager when it is necessary to contact a doctor about worsening asthma.

- Allow your child to recognize and avoid his or her asthma triggers.

TIPS FOR TEACHING YOUR FAMILY MEMBER ABOUT ASTHMA MEDICATIONS

Education is the key to asthma management. Here are some tips to follow when teaching your family member with asthma about his or her medications.

➤ If the prescription does not look right, consult your health care provider.

➤ Keep your medications in their original bottles. The original bottle has the correct label and instructions. Ask the pharmacist for an extra labeled container for when you travel.

➤ Do not substitute over-the-counter medications for the medications your doctor has prescribed.

➤ Most people with asthma and allergies can use over-the-counter decongestants and antihistamines safely.

➤ Ask your doctor about which decongestants and antihistamines are best for you.

➤ When your medications change, be sure to keep your old medications separate.

➤ When you first receive your medication, make sure the number of refills on the label matches the number on the original prescription.

➤ Contact your pharmacy well in advance of the time you need your medication. The pharmacist may need time to telephone the physician, check the medication supply, order the medication, then package and label the medication.

➤ Most prescriptions, including refills, are good for only 12 months. At that time, a new prescription is necessary, and any unused refills cannot be filled.

➤ Date the canister of your metered-dose inhaler so you know how long the medication lasts. Plan ahead to get the quantities you need.

➤ Note the expiration date on all medication packages.

➤ Make sure you check expiration dates on the medications you may have stored in different locations, such as at work or school or in your purse, backpack, or kitchen cabinet.

➤ Do not use any medications after they expire.

➤ Temperature changes and humidity can cause medications to become ineffective or dangerous.

➤ Humidity can cause a tablet to become moist and powdery. Do not store medications in places with high humidity, like a gym locker or the cabinet above the stove.

➤ Do not store medications in the glove compartment of your car. The temperature can range from −20°F to 120°F. When too cold or too hot, your metered-dose inhaler will not deliver a good spray and may burst. Check your metered-dose inhaler label for the recommended temperature range.

➤ When you travel, make sure you have a more than adequate supply of medications.

➤ Put your medications in your carry-on luggage.

➤ If there is more than one family member with asthma, instruct them not to share or exchange medications.

REMEMBERING TO TAKE MEDICATIONS

You should teach your family member with asthma and allergies to take his or her medications regularly. Here are two strategies you can use to foster regular medication use.

- Develop a daily routine for taking your medications. Pick something you do everyday, like waking, brushing your teeth, eating meals, or going to bed, and plan your medication schedule around that activity.

- Use a medication checklist or worksheet to record when you take medications. Place the checklist someplace visible as a reminder. (You can use stars or stickers on the chart for young children.)

Parents often want to prevent their child from having asthma attacks by putting limits on what the child can do. Remember that the goal of properly controlled asthma is to have a plan that lets the child do what he or she wants. This means not putting any limits on activities. You should strive to get your child's asthma under control so that he or she can take part in virtually all activities with other children. The goal is to treat your child with asthma as you would if he or she did not have this disease. The ideas in the list that follows may help you keep your child active and healthy.

1. Before setting any limits, look at what your child can already do. Then try to help your child do more. Do not make up rules that might hold him or her back without good reason.

2. Base any limits you set on what has really happened to your child. Do not base limits on what you think or fear might happen or on what might be true for other children with asthma. No two children with asthma are the same. Each child has different levels of physical fitness and maturity. Aim toward setting fewer or no limits and letting your child have more responsibility.

3. Discuss the limits you think are right for your child. Try to agree on limits that both of you can accept.

4. Discuss disagreements or doubts with your doctor so that he or she can help decide if these limits are necessary for your child.

5. Practice and review with your child those things that can help to manage an asthma attack if he or she accidentally goes beyond his or her limits.

6. To help your child do more, find specific ways to protect him or her from those things that can trigger an asthma attack. For example, if your child is allergic to animal dander and wants to visit a friend who has a dog, have your child take asthma medication before the visit or have the friend come to your house. Explain to your child that he or she should not pet or touch the animal and should leave the house if he or she feels an asthma attack coming on.

Single-Parenting the Child with Asthma

As we have seen, emotions are a significant asthma trigger. While stress does not cause asthma, it can precipitate an attack. Avoiding stress, just as you would another asthma trigger, is the best way to reduce its effects. In some instances, however, it is impossible to avoid stress. When divorce happens in a family, it can affect your child's asthma.

Divorce pulls the attention of parents from their child and his or her chronic condition to the emotional problems of a marital breakup. Young children with asthma need to feel that their parents are always monitoring their condition and are ready to respond should an attack strike. When parents are focused instead on marital problems, their child may feel that his or her asthma is no longer in the front of their minds. The divorce may also alter parents' viewpoint of their child's asthma. Parents may feel that a child is faking asthma attacks in order to gain attention or precipitate a reconciliation.

Add to these feelings the tremendous stress a divorce places on a household and you have the recipe for dangerous asthma. Children in this situation may be more likely to have an attack from other asthma triggers or from the overwhelming stress of the divorce.

If you are going through a divorce, take a few minutes to think about your child's asthma. Remember that with all the emotions during a divorce, it is possible to put your child's condition on the back burner. Try not to let your child's asthma care slip during this time. Trust your understanding of your child's asthma enough to know when he or she might be in real trouble from an attack.

If you do get divorced, you then have a new set of problems to deal with regarding your child's asthma—managing his or her condition as a single parent. If you and your spouse have separated or divorced, you are going to have to coordinate the care of your child with asthma. When a child moves between both parents' homes, it is easy for someone to get mixed up about his or her asthma medication schedule.

You should try to devise some strategy with your former spouse regarding your child's asthma care. If your child goes away for a weekend visit, prepare a list of the medications he or she receives regularly and the last time they were given. Talk with your former spouse about reporting regularly scheduled and rescue asthma medications used during the visit so that you can track your child's asthma management. And don't forget that there are now two homes that have to be free of asthma and allergy triggers.

Families with Asthma

Asthma and allergies are best managed in a partnership or co-management relationship that involves the family, the doctor, and other health care providers. This means involving family members in the care and management of the person with asthma and allergies. The family should operate as a team, with each member grounded in a basic understanding of asthma and allergies. Your family should understand how these conditions affect the person who has them and what medications and therapies can do to prevent and reverse attacks.

Families should band together to try to encourage members with asthma to follow their medical plan. Make sure your family:

- knows when to seek emergency care if a member has an attack

- understands the crisis plan in the event of a severe asthma attack

- knows and understands the treatment plan for helping a family member with asthma both on a regular basis and during a flare-up

- recognizes the family member's asthma warning signs so that the entire family can help with asthma care

- knows how to check the family member's asthma symptoms and peak flow readings to detect the early signs of an asthma attack

It's important for your family to participate in an asthma education program. Asthma education often includes lessons on such topics as what physical changes occur during an asthma attack, how to treat asthma with medications, how to manage stress, and how family and health care personnel can work with people with asthma to help them lead full lives. When the whole family is educated about asthma and allergies, your loved one with these conditions will live a fuller, more productive life. (If you are unable to participate in an education program, there are pamphlets, booklets, kits, and devices that you can use at home. And you can also encourage the entire family to read this book.)

Your entire family should be intimately familiar with asthma and allergy medications and how to use them. Properly used medications can prevent and reverse most asthma attacks. And in the case of an emergency, asthma medications can save a life. Your family should:

- learn about the medications the family member with asthma is taking
- know the brand name and generic name of the medications
- learn each medication's action, dose, when to take it, and what side effects to watch for
- understand any possible drug or food interactions

When the entire family learns about asthma and allergies and how to manage and control them, the person with asthma can rest assured that he or she is in good hands should an emergency happen.

13 / What to Tell the Baby-Sitter

YOU MAY ALREADY HAVE DISCOVERED THAT MOST BABY-SITTERS know little about asthma and allergies. Whether you are using a neighborhood teenager, grandparents, or a professional baby-sitting service, as a parent you are responsible for preparing the sitter to deal with your child's specific illness.

You should know that many professional sitter services do not want to get involved with the care of children with chronic diseases such as asthma and allergies. Fears stemming from concerns about liability and from inadequate knowledge about the conditions can frighten away many sitters. You may be able to overcome many of these concerns if you find a sitter with whom you are comfortable. It is important to remember that when preparing your child's sitter, you need to explain his or her complete asthma and allergy process.

The most important point to keep in mind when choosing a baby-sitter is to find a person who is willing to medicate and observe your child with asthma or allergies. Baby-sitters must be comfortable with administering medications to very young children or observing older children while they take their medications. For many prospective baby-sitters this would be a new task and something they are probably not familiar with. When interviewing prospective baby-sitters, it is important to determine if they are willing to handle medications.

If you find a baby-sitter whom you like and who is willing to medicate your child, it is probably less important that he or she already has knowledge about asthma and allergies. You can teach your baby-sitter enough about these illnesses to prepare him or her for caring for your child. But you cannot teach a baby-sitter who is unwilling or apprehensive about medications.

It is also critical that you find a baby-sitter who does not smoke. It is not enough to tell your child's sitter to smoke outside; you certainly do not want your child left unattended while the sitter is out having a cigarette. Nor do you want the sitter to take your child outside and be exposed to secondhand smoke. You should set hard-and-fast rules about smoking when your child is in the care of a sitter. This also applies to any guests the sitter may have over in your absence.

"Robby"

Ethan and Robin really have two baby-sitting experiences that stand out in their minds when they think of leaving their child, Robby, with a sitter. "The first time we left Robby with a sitter, it was a disaster," Robin says. "It was three years ago, when he was five, and it was the first time we had anyone but family watch him. We hired a very nice neighborhood teenager so that Ethan and I could go to the movies."

Robby's asthma was well under control, and he had never had trouble when he was left with his grandparents, so Ethan and Robin felt confident that everything would be fine. "We explained to the sitter that Robby had asthma, and we showed her his medications and how and when to use them," Ethan says. Then the couple left for the movies. "About halfway through the movie I had a feeling, so I called home," Robin says. "It turned out that Robby had been wheezing for half an hour and the sitter didn't know what to do. Ethan and I went straight home and managed to get his breathing under control by using the nebulizer. Robby was exhausted and the sitter was shattered," Robin says.

The couple put their son to bed and then tried to calm the nervous sitter. "We told her it wasn't her fault. I simply had not explained to her what to do in case of an emergency because we weren't expecting one," Ethan says. "I felt bad for her because she tried to do her best, but she just didn't have enough information and she was really nervous."

It was a year before Ethan and Robin tried again. They got the same teenage sitter, but this time sat down with her for half an hour and explained about Robby's condition, the triggers that could cause their son to have an attack, and what to do in case of an emergency. "I could tell she was a little nervous, but we told her she would be fine," Robin says. "I left her with an emergency plan that had the number of the restaurant Ethan and I were going to, our doctor's number, and the number of the local hospital. We also told her how to use Robby's inhaler with a spacer, because by now we had stopped using the nebulizer.

"Ethan and I had a nice dinner. We called twice during the evening and Robby was fine. He didn't have an attack that second time, but we felt much better knowing that if he had, our sitter would know what to do." ❑

Educating Your Baby-Sitter

Once you have found a caring, nurturing baby-sitter who is not afraid of medicating your child, you must train the sitter about asthma and allergies and about your child's specific disease process. Remember that baby-sitters do not have to become as expert in the disease as you or your child. But they do have to know enough about the condition to recognize the warning signs of an attack and to take action to reverse your child's flare-up. It is a good idea to start by giving your baby-sitter a brief overview of these conditions and how they work in the body.

Your child's baby-sitter needs to know that asthma is a chronic condition that leaves airways inflamed and prone to constrict, thus making it hard for your child to breathe. The baby-sitter should know that your child's airways are more likely to constrict when he or she is exposed to some asthma trigger. Your baby-sitter should be familiar with the asthma and allergy triggers that can cause your child to have an attack. It is a good idea to leave your baby-sitter a list of these triggers, including any foods that should be avoided. You can use the sample sheet, Instructions for the Baby-Sitter, at the end of this chapter, to give the baby-sitter all the information needed to properly manage your child's disease.

The baby-sitter should know that asthma is a real condition and not the result of some emotional or psychological problem. The more baby-sitters know about your child's illness, the more apt they are to remain calm if your child's disease flares up while you are away. You should explain how important it is to remain calm during an asthma attack and how excitement can worsen the attack. If your child is old enough to control his or her own disease, explain to the baby-sitter that your child has been taught to remain calm during an attack.

You must also educate your sitter about your child's medications. If you have a young child who is using a nebulizer, the sitter needs to be taught how to use the device. Older children who are using an inhaler with a spacer and face mask require less attention, but the sitter should still know how these devices work. In addition to any regularly scheduled medications, you should tell the sitter about any inhaled asthma medications, such as beta-adrenergic drugs, your child uses during an asthma attack. The sitter should know how much of these emergency medications your child can use before his or her condition warrants seeking medical attention.

Teach your child's sitter about the warning signs of an impending asthma attack. The sitter should be able to recognize that your child may be having an attack if he or she is coughing, wheezing, having difficulty breathing, or sucking in his or her chest. Leave your sitter with a plan of action that must be followed in case of an attack. (You can use the following sample plans and tailor them to your specific needs.)

EMERGENCY ASTHMA PLAN FOR YOUNGER CHILDREN

If you notice my child displaying any of the signs of an asthma attack, begin the following treatment with the nebulizer:

Put _____ drops of _____ in the unit. Attach the face mask to his/her face and turn the nebulizer on. You should leave the nebulizer on for _____ minutes, even if it appears that my child is breathing easier.

If his/her breathing does not ease within 3 to 5 minutes, call me immediately. I can be reached at _____.

If you cannot reach me, or if my child's breathing gets worse, call his/her doctor.
Dr. _____ Phone: _____

If you cannot reach the doctor, or if the doctor recommends taking my child to the hospital, please take him/her immediately to _____ hospital. Bring a list of the medications he/she has taken during the evening and our health insurance information, which is located _____

_____.

You may also want to leave your sitter with a simple checklist of do's and don'ts to minimize the chance that your child will have an attack in your absence and to ensure that an attack can be properly managed should one strike. Your list should take into account your own child's disease pattern. The following list is a good starting point that you can add to or delete items from to suit your child's needs.

- Do make my child aware that you understand he/she has asthma or allergies and know what to do in case of an emergency.

- Do make sure my child uses his/her regularly scheduled medications on time.

- Do try to reduce my child's exposure to the asthma and allergy triggers that can cause him/her to have an attack.

EMERGENCY ASTHMA PLAN FOR OLDER CHILDREN

If you notice my child displaying any of the signs of an asthma attack, ask him/her if he/she is having trouble breathing. My child knows enough about his/her disease to recognize when he/she needs medications.

He/she can take _____ puffs of the _____ inhaler.

If his/her breathing does not ease within 3 to 5 minutes, call me immediately. I can be reached at _____.

If you cannot reach me, or if my child's breathing gets worse, call his/her doctor.
Dr. _____ Phone: _____

If you cannot reach the doctor, or if the doctor recommends taking my child to the hospital, please take him/her immediately to _____ hospital. Bring a list of the medications he/she has taken during the evening and our health insurance information, which is located _____

_____.

- Do watch for any signs of an impending asthma attack.

- Do ask my child if he/she is having trouble breathing if you see any of the signs of an impending attack.

- Do use the emergency asthma medications I have left for you if my child has an attack.

- Do call me if his/her breathing does not get better after using these medications.

- Do call our family doctor or the hospital if you cannot reach me.

- Don't baby my child or treat him/her differently because he/she has asthma and allergies.

- Don't let him/her get away with behavior otherwise considered unacceptable.

- Don't worry. My child's disease is under control and he/she knows what to do in case of breathing problems.

- Don't get excited if he/she has trouble breathing.

- Don't hesitate to call me or our doctor if you think there is trouble.

INSTRUCTIONS FOR THE BABY-SITTER

Sitter: _____

Child: _____ Age: _____

Child: _____ Age: _____

Child: _____ Age: _____

_____ has asthma and takes the following medications on a regular basis:

_____ Next dose to be given at: _____

_____ Next dose to be given at: _____

_____ Next dose to be given at: _____

The triggers that can cause my child to have an asthma or allergy attack are:

_____

_____

_____

_____

_____

You should try to see that he/she avoids exposure to these allergens and triggers.

My child also takes the following medication when he/she is wheezing or having trouble breathing. He/she should use no more than _____ puffs over the next _____ hours.

If you notice that my child is wheezing, struggling to breathe, coughing, or inhaling so hard that he/she is sucking in his/her chest, it is time to give the above medication. If that medication does not work to ease breathing, he/she may need medical attention. It is important for you to remain calm during an asthma attack, as any sign of nervousness on your part may cause my child to become nervous and his/her asthma attack to worsen.

You can reach me at: _____.

If I am unable to be reached, contact: _____

or _____.

If you cannot reach me, or if after talking to me we decide my child needs medical attention, call his/her doctor.

Dr. _____ Phone: _____

In case of an emergency, take my child to the local hospital for immediate asthma care.

Hospital: _____ Phone: _____

Health Insurance: _____ ID#: _____

Leaving your child with asthma and allergies in the care of someone else can be an anxious experience. But if your child is educated about his or her disease and you have left the baby-sitter with enough information about how to manage your child's disease and what to do in case of an emergency, you will be able to enjoy a night out knowing that your child is in good hands.

14 / What to Tell the School

FOR PARENTS AROUND THE COUNTRY, THE END OF THE SUMMER means one thing—preparing for the return to school. From new clothes to lunch boxes to notebooks and pencil cases, parents and children busy themselves for the start of the new school year. For the parents of children with asthma and allergies, however, adequately preparing for the start of the school year requires more than outfitting their child with the latest fashions. The child also needs to be outfitted with his or her latest medication schedule, emergency asthma plan, and letters informing teachers, school nurses, and administrators of any special needs.

The start of the school year means that your child with asthma and allergies will be spending the better part of the day away from your watchful eyes, by now the eyes that are probably the most trained to spot the early signs of an asthma or allergy attack. That does not have to mean your child will be away from proper asthma or allergy management. Parents need to educate their children about their disease. Teach them to understand the signs of an impending attack, instruct them on how to use their medications, and make them knowledgeable about the asthma and allergy triggers to which they are sensitive. Armed with this information, children can largely take over their disease management while at school.

Make sure your child's teachers, school nurses, administrators, and physical education instructors are aware of his or her condition. Most school officials have encountered children with asthma and allergies before. Nevertheless, you should inform them of your child's specific problems and disease management plan in detail.

Advance Planning for Your Child

Before school starts, find out about any forms the school may require for children who use medications while at school. Bring the completed forms to school officials so that you can have a face-to-face visit about your child's condition.

Approach this meeting as a chance for mutual learning. You want to learn about the school's policies on medication use and its experience with children with asthma and allergies. At the same time you want school officials to learn about your child's specific and unique disease characteristics. During this meeting you should:

- make certain that school officials understand that asthma is a real condition and that it is neither contagious nor psychological.

- explain your child's medication schedule. If he or she takes regular medications to prevent asthma attacks, make that clear and distinguish between these medications and others your child may need to control attacks of wheezing.

- point out that if your child is wheezing or is short of breath at rest, he or she requires the immediate use of the inhaler or liquid medication you use to reverse acute asthma attacks. Explain that your child has been taught to remain calm during an attack, so teachers need to pay attention to his or her request for an inhaler even if he or she seems calm and relaxed.

- remind school administrators that they should remain calm during an attack. Explain that your child knows what to do and that it is important not to get excited, as this may cause your child to become anxious and escalate the attack.

- list your child's asthma and allergy triggers and ask that this list be distributed to all your child's instructors. Common triggers in schools include dust and dust mites, class pets, plants, certain chemicals used in science classes, particles and fumes from construction, pollens and mold spores, and exercise.

- provide the asthma and allergy medications your child uses and note that you will refill these products as needed.

- leave a peak flow meter identical to the one your child uses at home. It's a good idea to mark your child's normal and trouble zone ranges on the meter.

- bring a copy of your child's asthma emergency management plan that you developed with your child's doctor. Make sure your child's teachers and the school nurse are familiar with the plan.

- bring all information regarding any history or risk your child may have for anaphylaxis from insect stings or other allergens. Make sure the school administrators know what anaphylaxis is, that it can be quite serious, and that immediate medical attention is required.

- leave an anaphylaxis emergency kit with the school nurse if your child has this risk. Make sure the nurse knows how to use this kit and point out that the kit needs to be taken on class trips your child attends.

While many school nurses have training in asthma and allergy care, unfortunately most schools do not employ full-time school nurses. Many rely on volunteers or aides trained in first aid and simple medical procedures. It is up to you to make sure that the people at the school who are in charge of your child's asthma and allergy care are familiar with the disease and know the specifics of your child's case. Nothing is too simplistic to go over when your child's health is at stake. A face-to-face meeting in which you provide needed information is important in establishing a good relationship with the people who will have charge of your child for a large part of his or her day.

For your meeting with school officials, it is a good idea to provide letters outlining your child's disease, any medications he or she may be taking, and what you expect from the school to help in the management of your child's disease. The following pages contain 2 sample letters you can use, one for the school nursing office and one for your child's teachers.

Even with the best of planning, your child may suffer an asthma attack while at school. That is why, in the list above, you are advised to provide the school with the emergency asthma management plan developed with your doctor. This plan should list your child's best peak flow reading and readings that indicate the beginnings of a problem. Also on this plan are what medications the child should take in the event of an attack and when your child may need to see a doctor or go to a hospital. (For a sample asthma emergency plan, see chapter 5.)

Asthma and Allergy Triggers in the School

Schools can be wonderful places of learning and discovery, but they can also be home to many common asthma and allergy triggers. The most common trigger in schools is physical exercise. Whether or not your child has exercise-induced asthma, many factors can trigger an attack during gym class. If the activity is held outdoors, the cold, dry air during certain seasons can irritate your child's airways, causing constriction and wheezing. Children may also overexert themselves during competition, leading to a potential attack.

INFORMATION FOR THE SCHOOL NURSE

My child, _____, has asthma. In most circumstances this condition does not stop him/her from participating in activities with the rest of the class. He/she should not have activities restricted because of this condition. However, there are occasions when his/her asthma may flare up. During an asthma flare-up he/she should not go out in the cold or participate in strenuous physical activity.

My child must take the following medications during school at the hours noted to control his/her condition (check those that apply):

____ theophylline, _____ mg, at _____.

____ cromolyn, _____ puffs, at _____.

____ inhaled steroids, _____ puffs, at _____.

____ inhaled beta-adrenergics, _____ puffs, at _____.

____ He/she also uses an inhaler before sports and if wheezing during physical activity.

____ He/she should carry his/her inhaler at all times, ____ leave it in the locker, ____ leave it in the health room.

____ My child understands his/her disease and how to manage it. He/she knows when he/she needs to use an inhaler; please let him/her determine when this is necessary. He/she is not to use the inhaled beta-adrenergic drug more than once a day unless an emergency arises or I write you a note.

Please let me know if I can provide you with more information regarding my child's condition or medications. Attached you will find the emergency asthma care plan developed by my child's doctor in case of an emergency.

If you have any questions, please call me at home, _____, or at work, _____.

If you can't reach me, please call _____, who is apprised of my child's condition, or our physician, Dr. _____, at _____.

Sincerely,

_____

INFORMATION FOR TEACHERS

My child, _____, has asthma. Ordinarily, this condition does not stop him/her from participating in school activities, nor should he/she be restricted in any way because of this condition. He/she may have an occasional asthma flare-up. If this happens, he/she should not go out in the cold or participate in strenuous physical activity.

The school health staff know about this condition and the medication my child needs to take regularly and during an asthma attack. My child has been taught to remain calm during an attack, but do not think his/her calm demeanor means he/she can go without treatment if he/she says it is needed. He/she understands this condition and knows what to do in case of an asthma attack.

Please allow my child to go retrieve his/her inhaler and use it when he/she feels it is necessary. If you feel he/she is abusing this privilege, please let me know.

A list of my child's medications has been left with the school health department. Some of these medications can cause headaches, stomach upset, or make him/her restless and jumpy. However, he/she should not be allowed to misbehave more than any other child in the class, and I want to know of any discipline problems my child creates.

If you have any questions or concerns, I would be more than happy to discuss them with you.

Sincerely,

_____

You should meet with your child's physical education instructor and inform him or her about your child's condition. Explain that asthma or allergies alone do not prevent your child from taking part in all the activities that other children perform. Tell the instructor that you do not want your child excluded from sports simply because he or she has asthma. But it is important that the instructor know that if your child does experience wheezing or breathing difficulty, he or she must be excused to use medications immediately. Most children with asthma can return to physical education once their medications have reversed their wheezing. (A discussion of the effects of exercise on asthma appears in chapter 15.)

Dust and dust mites are often a problem in schools because it is difficult to keep classrooms and bookshelves free of these potential asthma and allergy triggers. Dust and dust mites can also exist in day care and preschool settings, so you may want to provide an encased pillow or an allergy-free cover for your child's pillow for use during nap or quiet times.

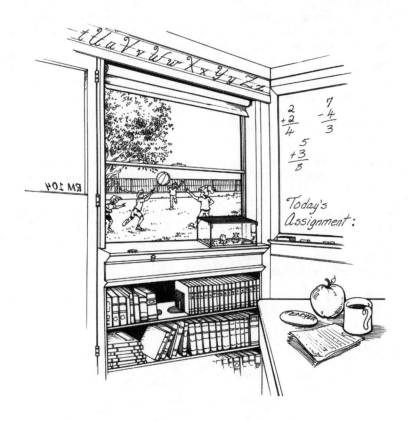

Dusty books, laboratory animals, chalk dust, and allergen-filled schoolyards all can pose problems at school for children with allergies.

Cockroaches are another big asthma trigger in school buildings. Roaches may be attracted to lunches kept in lockers or to food in the school's kitchen. As discussed in chapter 3, cockroaches are a potent asthma and allergy trigger that can cause asthma attacks and lead to inflammation in the airways that can result in future attacks. Urge your school administrators to fumigate the school regularly and clean the grounds of dead roaches.

The science class is often a home to asthma and allergy triggers. White rats, gerbils, guinea pigs, or other furry animals can play havoc with your child's asthma. Determine if your child's science class has any live animal pets. If so, ask your doctor if your child can take any medications before class to reduce the chance that these asthma and allergy triggers will lead to an attack. Often a preventive dose of inhaled cromolyn or beta-adrenergic drugs can stave off a wheezing attack for the hour or so that your child will be around these animals. If your child has allergies, ask your doctor about a nonsedating antihistamine or a nasal version of cromolyn or a steroid to prevent the misery of an allergic reaction. These medications are described in detail in earlier chapters. By employing some preventive medication maintenance, your child with asthma and allergies should be able to attend science class as usual. If your child has severe disease, you may need to talk with the science teacher about excusing him or her from the few classes a year in which there are live animals present.

Chalk dust, odors from harsh industrial cleaners, fumes from epoxy and other building materials, and particles from construction all have the potential of triggering your child's asthma and allergies. You can't rid your child's school of all these triggers, but by talking with your child about what was happening when he or she had an attack at school, you can narrow down what is triggering his or her asthma at school. Armed with that knowledge, you may then be able to take steps to reduce your child's exposure to the offending trigger.

When Your Child Should Stay Home

It is often difficult to determine when the child with asthma needs to miss school. By setting up good communication lines with school officials and teachers, you may be able to reduce the number of days your child misses school because of asthma. If school officials and teachers are well informed about your child's asthma, you may be able to send him or her off to school even on days when there are hints of a problem. Even under the best of circumstances, however, there are times when a child with asthma may need to miss school. Here are some guidelines to follow when deciding whether your child should attend school.

Your child can probably go to school if he or she:

- has a stuffy or runny nose but is not wheezing
- has a mild wheeze that clears up with medication before heading off to school
- feels he or she can perform most of the usual activities
- is not having trouble breathing

Your child should stay home if he or she:

- is having difficulty breathing
- is wheezing and the wheezing does not clear up after medications are given
- has any of the signs of an asthma attack, such as breathing faster than usual, laboring for each breath, and sucking in so hard to fill the lungs that his or her chest appears concave
- has evidence of an infection, sore throat, or swollen glands
- has a fever or feels hot and flushed
- is so weak or tired it will be hard to take part in typical activities
- has such severe allergy symptoms, such as a runny nose, itchy, watery eyes, and a cough, that it would be hard to take part in usual activities

If you decide that your child's asthma or allergy flare-up is so severe that it requires staying home from school, don't let the occasion cause your child to get behind in schoolwork. This is especially true if your child must miss more than a day of classes. Contact your child's teachers, explain the situation, and ask if there is any homework your child can do to keep up with the class. While making up missed work at home can be difficult when your child is having an asthma attack, a little patience can help him or her keep up to speed.

This approach has numerous positive effects. Although your child must miss school, he or she will have less to catch up with upon returning to class. By performing work even when home, children develop a sense of self-esteem, knowing that while asthma may cause them to miss an occasional school day, it does not mean they must fall behind in their studies. And it will ensure that your child does not begin using asthma as an excuse to stay home. After all, when given the choice between doing work at home with parents or doing it at school with friends and all the distractions of the school day, most children will choose the latter.

Open Airways For Schools

To better educate children, parents, school administrators, nurses, teachers, and physical education instructors about asthma, the American Lung Association has adopted and implemented the Open Airways For Schools program. The program is used as a teaching aid to help children understand what asthma is, how it affects breathing, and how it can be controlled. Children learn through the use of role playing, storytelling, games, artistic expression, and physical activities meant to show how to control the panicky feelings when an asthma attack strikes.

A PARENT'S CHECKLIST

❑ Educate child so he/she is capable of managing his/her own disease while at school.

❑ Talk with school administrators and individual teachers about your child's asthma.

❑ Explain that your child understands his/her condition and can manage the disease successfully.

❑ Make sure teachers understand the need for your child to use his/her inhaler when he/she feels it is necessary.

❑ Determine school policy about having child keep asthma inhalers on school grounds.

❑ Present asthma emergency plan, peak flow meter, and asthma drugs to the school health staff for young children or in schools that mandate such a procedure.

❑ Make sure your child always has an anaphylaxis emergency kit on hand with a spare kept in the school health department if he/she is at risk for this severe form of allergy.

❑ Send letters explaining your child's condition to school administrators, nurses, and teachers.

❑ Talk with school officials about strategies to reduce asthma and allergy triggers, especially animals in science classes and cockroaches.

❑ Talk with the physical education instructor about your child's asthma and the few instances in which he/she may need to be excused or take part in less strenuous activities.

❑ Request that work be sent home when your child misses school due to asthma.

❑ Explain the American Lung Association's Open Airways For Schools program and urge school administrators to take part in the program.

❑ Offer to call the local American Lung Association chapter and have Open Airways For Schools information forwarded to the school's principal.

"Mark"

Mark has had asthma since he was three years old. Growing up with the condition, he became quite adept at managing the disease himself. And before his family moved, Mark was able to do just that. He uses an inhaled steroid three times a day and has a beta-adrenergic inhaler for attacks of wheezing. At his old school he kept his asthma inhalers with him or in his desk during school and used them only when necessary. But in the eighth grade Mark's family moved to a new neighborhood in a new school district. Mark's mother, Beth, went to the new school to tell the principal and teachers about Mark's condition but found that the new school's policy was that Mark had to leave his asthma medications in the school health office.

"I tried to explain to them that Mark has been controlling his own disease for years, but they said it was school policy that all medications be kept in the health department," Beth says. Beth was told that Mark could go down to the health department when he needed to use his steroid inhaler and whenever he felt it was necessary to use the beta-adrenergic drug. Beth sent letters to all of Mark's teachers and dropped off his medications and asthma emergency plan with the health department.

For a while everything was fine. Mark regularly went to the health department to use his steroid inhaler and, whenever he was wheezing, to use the beta-adrenergic inhaler. But one Friday during gym class, Mark began to wheeze. He asked the physical education instructor if he could go to the health department to use his spray, and the instructor said no. "He thought I was just trying to skip out on class because I had done that before, but this time I was really starting to get into trouble," Mark says. Clearly wheezing now, he asked the instructor again, but because the instructor was busy, he didn't notice Mark's condition and once again said no.

"I knew I had to do something, so I just got up and left," Mark says. "I was afraid of what he was going to do, but I knew I needed my inhaler." The instructor started yelling at Mark as he left gym class, but Mark made a beeline for the health department. He was wheezing when he entered the door, and the nurse immediately gave him his inhaler. Around the time that Mark's wheezing was settling down, the physical education instructor came into the room. "As soon as he came in, he could see that I hadn't been faking and he apologized," Mark says.

"When Mark came home and told me, I was so mad I wanted to go right down there and start yelling at that instructor," Beth says. "But then I realized it must be hard for these teachers to know when kids are just trying to get out of their class and when the few with asthma are really having an attack. So I calmed down and wrote a very nice letter to the principal explaining what had happened and noting that I understood the troubles that the teachers have. I also wrote that Mark had told me he had skipped class for no reason before, that I was going to discipline him for that, and that I wanted to know if Mark ever abused his privileges to go to the health department. But the most important thing was to get the principal to explain to all of Mark's teachers that they have to take his attacks seriously and let him use his medications as soon as he thinks it is necessary."

Beth says that the principal wrote back explaining that he had talked to all of Mark's teachers and made them aware of his condition. The principal said Mark would not be stopped from using his medications again. ❏

In the Open Airways For Schools program, children with asthma learn how to recognize the warning signs of an attack, are taught the management steps they need to control their disease, and learn about the effects asthma has on their lungs. Each activity is designed so it can be incorporated into the daily classroom schedule.

The program comes with instructions for teachers, school administrators, nurses, and physical education instructors, which explain asthma in simple terms, give tips on how students with asthma can be better managed, and include sample medical forms to track children with asthma. If you want your child's school to participate in the Open Airways For Schools program, tell your child's principal or school administrator. The program can be obtained from your local chapter of the American Lung Association (1–800–LUNG–USA).

15 / The Benefits of Exercise

EXERCISE MAY BE THE ONE TRUE FOUNTAIN OF YOUTH. Regular exercise has been shown to lead to weight loss, a better-conditioned heart, stronger muscles, and a more active, vibrant lifestyle. The benefits of exercise hold true even for people with asthma and allergies. Regular exercise can lead to better conditioning and less shortness of breath during strenuous activities. Most people with asthma and allergies can exercise as much as desired, and doctors recommend you take advantage of this ability to condition your heart, lungs, and entire body.

For years it was thought that people with asthma could not and should not take part in team sports and vigorous activities. We now know that this was a fallacy; most people with well-controlled asthma can participate in regular physical activities and exercise programs with minimal difficulties. Today, with proper detection and treatment, those affected by asthma are capable of exercise that's beneficial to both their physical health and their emotional well-being.

Despite the benefits of regular exercise, many people with asthma and allergies avoid working out. Some may fear having an attack; others may have bad memories of an asthma flare-up during past exercise; and still others may feel out of shape because of their disease and embarrassed to begin a program. A vicious cycle is often seen in people with breathing problems. People with asthma may feel breathless or show other signs of asthma at lower levels of activity than people with normal lungs. To avoid this sensation, they may reduce their level of activity, which leads to a greater degree of deconditioning, which in turn increases breathlessness at even lower levels of exercise. This can be especially true among children with asthma, for whom the cycle may continue through adolescence and into adulthood.

Regular exercise is critical for everyone with asthma, but it is especially important for children and teens. Many habits are well formed by the time people reach their early teens. Children with asthma who shun exercise may learn to avoid outdoor play, sports, and other physical activities that can produce asthma symptoms. Untreated asthma can limit normal activities; this may result in lasting physical and psychological effects, including poor self-image. And because of their decreased participation, children with asthma may be considered lazy. (Parents who want their child with asthma to participate in school sports and activities should refer to chapter 14 for tips on how to approach coaches and physical education instructors about their child's breathing condition.)

Exercise-Induced Asthma

People with asthma and allergies should be aware of some potential problems before undertaking an exercise regimen. The most important is a condition known as exercise-induced asthma, which is very common among people with asthma. Eighty to 90 percent of asthma sufferers have difficulty breathing during vigorous exercise. The condition even affects a number of people who have not been diagnosed with asthma but develop breathing problems during vigorous exercise — for example, 50 percent of people with allergic rhinitis and 10 percent of athletes with normal lung function have been found to develop exercise-induced asthma.

Exercise-induced asthma is a temporary narrowing of the airways, or bronchospasm, that is induced by strenuous exercise. Doctors are not completely sure how exercise triggers asthma, nor do they completely understand how exercise can induce bronchospasm in people who do not have asthma. But they do have some theories. During vigorous exercise the body requires more oxygen. This increased oxygen demand causes us to breathe at a faster rate, which causes our airways to become cool and dry. For people with asthma, who already have inflamed, hyperresponsive airways, this cooling and drying effect can act as an asthma trigger. In fact, it may be that the large intake of cool, dry air stimulates mast cells to release the chemicals that trigger an asthma attack in the same way that smoke, pollen, and other asthma triggers work on the mast cells.

Doctors believe that the cooling of the airways, combined with a loss of water from the airways that occurs during exercise, is responsible for many exercise-induced asthma attacks. Breathing warm, humidified air, such as the air inhaled during swimming, can completely or partially prevent exercise-induced asthma, whereas breathing cold, dry air seems to make exercise-induced asthma symptoms worse for many people.

ATHLETES WITH ASTHMA

Asthma doesn't stop many of the world's most elite athletes from exercising, competing, and even setting world records and winning Olympic medals. Hundreds of athletes with asthma compete in sports as varied as track and field, swimming, and cross-country skiing. Even a short list of the world's premier athletes with asthma is dotted with impressive names and accomplishments. All of the following athletes have asthma but haven't let it stop them from fulfilling their dreams.

• Debby Myers won three Olympic gold medals in swimming in 1964.

• Rick Dumont won the gold in the 1500-meter swim at the 1976 Olympic games.

• Jackie Joyner-Kersee won gold medals for the heptathlon in 1988 and 1992 and the long jump in 1988, as well as bronze medals for the long jump in 1992 and 1996.

• Professional basketball players Danny Manning of the Los Angeles Clippers, Mike Jiminsky of the Philadelphia 76ers, and Sam Perkins of the Dallas Mavericks play with asthma.

• Rosa Mota won Olympic gold in the marathon for Portugal at the 1988 games.

• Mike Storm won a silver medal in the pentathlon at the 1984 games.

• Countless others, from track and field star Evelyn Ashford to professional dancer Christine Dakin of the Martha Graham Company to triathlete Cheryl Decker, give their best to the sports they love.

Around the world, athletes with asthma compete regularly despite numerous restrictions from athletic committees on the types of drugs they can use to control their asthma. The International Olympic Committee bans the use of epinephrine-type drugs to control wheezing and coughing and certain decongestants, such as those containing ephedrine, because the committee believes that these drugs may also enhance performance. Inhaled steroids like cromolyn sodium, anticholinergics, and theophylline are allowed, as are many of today's inhaled beta-adrenergic drugs.

If these athletes can overcome their disease even with the restrictions on the types of medications they can use, so can you. Take it from the top athletes in the world: asthma is no reason to shy away from exercising.

Exercise-induced asthma can cause symptoms similar to asthma attacks triggered by other substances. The most obvious are wheezing, shortness of breath on exertion, and chest tightness. Most people who have these types of symptoms when exercising have been diagnosed as having asthma; they take medications regularly, and they generally have symptoms when exposed to other asthma triggers. Some people, however, can develop less obvious asthma symptoms from exercise. These can include coughing (for instance, a person may consistently cough after jogging or playing basketball or soccer), chest congestion, chest tightness or pain, shortness of breath, susceptibility to cold air (consistent coughing after coming in from outside in winter), feeling out of shape or winded, tiring easily, lack of energy (especially in children), or problems that occur while running but not while swimming.

Parents have to be especially sharp-eyed to spot some cases of exercise-induced asthma in children. You should suspect this condition if your child is unable to keep up with his or her friends when running and playing, cannot run for five minutes without stopping, or gets dizzy or develops stomachaches when exercising. Because many people become winded when they exercise, many parents, physicians, teachers, and even the children themselves overlook the signs of exercise-induced asthma. But parents should become keenly aware of the signs and train their children to recognize them. Wheezing after exercising is far more serious than simply becoming out of breath from working up a good sweat, and people with asthma should take steps to prevent reactions to this asthma trigger in the same way they address exposure to other asthma triggers.

Stages of Exercise-Induced Asthma

Exercise-induced asthma appears to occur in three stages. The early phase, which is also the most severe, generally occurs following 6 to 8 minutes of vigorous exercise, peaks at 5 to 10 minutes after exercise, and lasts 30 to 60 minutes after the activity has stopped. During this time people with asthma experience the typical signs of asthma, such as wheezing and coughing. The symptoms can become so severe that the affected person must stop exercising and take medications to reverse the attack.

This first stage of exercise-induced asthma is considered especially dangerous because it can be difficult to treat even if you stop exercising. That is because the airways may remain cool and dry for 15 to

30 minutes after you stop exercising, exposing your airways to the asthma trigger even after you think you have reduced your exposure.

It is during this early phase that doctors are best able to measure your reaction to exercise. If you have frequent bouts of exercise-induced asthma, your doctor may ask you to take a test of your lung function after walking on a treadmill to simulate exercise. Doctors can measure the amount of airway obstruction during an exercise-induced attack by gauging how quickly air can be exhaled in the first second before and after 6 to 8 minutes of vigorous exercise. This can help determine the severity of the asthma or the exercise-induced asthma.

After the initial bout of exercise-induced asthma, there may be a period of 30 to 90 minutes during which little or no wheezing or other symptoms are present. This refractory period, as it is called, happens to about 50 percent of people with exercise-induced asthma. Athletes with exercise-induced asthma may routinely take advantage of this refractory period to allow themselves to compete. Some athletes with exercise-induced asthma time an initial workout so that they will be in this symptom-free second phase when it is time to compete. Some athletes find that if they run a long distance even after becoming symptomatic in the first phase, they can actually run through their bronchospasm into the second phase.

This second, symptom-free phase may be the result of chemicals that are released during exercise that serve to relax and widen the airways. Unless you have very well controlled asthma, are in excellent physical shape, and know precisely how exercise affects your asthma, you should not try this approach. It is better that you follow the steps on page 187 to prevent and treat exercise-induced asthma than to continue working out when you are wheezing. Finally, some people have a late-phase response to exercise, which can begin 12 to 16 hours after exercise has stopped. Doctors feel these late-phase reactions are typically the easiest to treat.

Factors That Influence Exercise-Induced Asthma

Several important factors, including how well your asthma is controlled, the conditions under which you exercise, and the type of exercise, can influence the onset and severity of exercise-induced asthma. As we have seen, asthma can be controlled in most cases. When your asthma is under good control, you will be virtually symptom free, even during exercise. But people with poorly controlled asthma are prone to more attacks from all asthma triggers, including exercise. The more inflammation present in the airways, the more hypersensitive, or "twitchy," the airways and the more likely that even minimal exercise can cause exercise-induced asthma attacks.

If a person with asthma has difficulty breathing during even the lightest exercise, the asthma is probably not being properly controlled. This may be especially evident in children who regularly have difficulty keeping up in gym class or in team sports. Exercise tolerance is in fact an excellent measure of whether or not asthma is under good control. If you find that asthma is preventing you or your child from exercising, you should see your doctor. It may be that a change in medications is required until the inflammation is treated and symptoms are relieved. (Treating and preventing exercise-induced asthma is discussed later in this chapter.)

As we have seen, most people with asthma are prone to exercise-induced attacks. This is the case even when your asthma is under good control from medications that reduce the underlying inflammation in your airways. The body's oxygen needs are increased during exercise, and this increased need translates into faster and harder breathing. When people with asthma breathe harder and faster, they not only cause cooling and drying of the airways but they may inhale more asthma and allergy triggers.

Exercising in the presence of numerous asthma triggers can therefore increase the chance that you will suffer an exercise-induced attack. The following asthma triggers can work to heighten or trigger an exercise-induced asthma attack. If you are prone to exercise-induced asthma, doctors recommend that you try not to exercise:

- in cold, dry air (outside or indoors)
- outside in the winter
- outside when air pollution indexes are high
- on freshly cut grass or when levels of tree and weed pollens are high
- in overly dusty gyms
- around people wearing strongly scented perfumes or cosmetics
- when you are still getting over a recent cold or asthma attack
- if you are overly tired
- if you feel unusually stressed

The type and intensity of your workout can also determine if you will get an asthma attack from exercising. Exercise-induced asthma is most often brought on by aerobic sports, such as those that require continuous and long-lasting exercise that results in deep and rapid breathing. Running, cross-country skiing, cycling, aerobics classes, and soccer are examples of activities that require continuous or near continuous activity. Doctors believe that intermittent high anaerobic activity is preferable to sustained long-duration aerobic activity for people with asthma. Circuit training, in which a person switches activities every five minutes or so, is a good example of an asthma-friendly exercise.

Choosing the Best Exercise

While there is no such thing as the perfect exercise for people with exercise-induced asthma, some activities do appear better than others. The key is to select a sport or exercise you enjoy and feel good about doing. Indoor swimming, because it is performed in a humid and often warm environment, and very light or nonaerobic exercise, such as walking or weight training, rarely result in exercise-induced asthma. Running tends to produce symptoms more easily than do bicycling or walking. Exercise intensity should begin at low levels and gradually increase as your fitness level improves.

Low- and High-Risk Exercises for People with Asthma

Sports and activities *less* likely to trigger asthma	
Football	Volleyball
Tennis	Wrestling
Baseball	Weight lifting
Golf	Swimming
Gymnastics	Short-distance track and field events

Sports and activities *more* likely to trigger asthma	
Running	Aerobics
Cross-country skiing	Soccer
Cycling	

When deciding on exercise, the most important factor is to pick something you are comfortable with. People with asthma find that certain activities are more likely than others to cause asthma attacks, but whether any given exercise routine will trigger an attack is individual. The best approach is to try different routines and determine what is the best for you. For instance, while running may be more likely to trigger attacks in many people with asthma, you may find that you are able to jog moderately without any trouble. Virtually all people with asthma can exercise regularly without fear of an attack if they slowly work up to their potential. There is no substitute for good judgment.

Ways to Reduce Exercise-Induced Asthma

If you have asthma symptoms when exercising, there are some simple things you can do to reduce the chance you will have an exercise-induced attack. First and foremost, you should avoid exercise if you have any indication of breathing difficulties before starting. Even the slightest wheeze can turn into an attack when you increase your exposure to any asthma trigger.

Before beginning your exercise routine, you should warm up your body and muscles. This is sound advice for anyone before exercising and will also reduce your chance of an asthma attack. Try walking and other low-level aerobic activities, stretching exercises, and running rapidly in place for 30 seconds, followed by a 60-second rest. Repeat this routine two or three times before starting your exercise program.

As always, you should try to reduce your exposure to other asthma and allergy triggers. Inhaled allergens, such as dust and dust mites, pollens, animal dander, and air pollutants, are all known to aggravate exercise-induced asthma. People with inhaled allergies may find exercise more difficult in places where these triggers are present. You should try to exercise in places that have low quantities of asthma triggers, or you may need to take a preventive dose of asthma medications before beginning your exercise regimen. Try to minimize your outside exercise time when it is cold, and if you do work out in such weather, try wearing a scarf or cold-air mask to warm and moisten the air before it reaches your airways. When you have finished exercising, do not stop suddenly. This could cause the temperature and humidity in your airways to change abruptly, possibly leading to an attack. Take at least a 10-minute cool-down period composed of light aerobics and stretching.

Treating Exercise-Induced Asthma

Fortunately, there is a simple and effective way of treating exercise-induced asthma. By following a prescribed "pretreatment plan," people with asthma should be able to participate safely and successfully in exercise, sports, and other physical activities. Pretreatment with certain asthma medications can prevent exercise from triggering asthma symptoms. Many people who have well-controlled asthma but experience asthma symptoms during exercise respond well to the use of an inhaled short-acting beta-adrenergic medication, such as albuterol. This medication is usually prescribed to be taken 10 to 15 minutes before exercise and quickly opens the airways to prevent asthma symptoms. Some people with exercise-induced asthma respond well to other medications; using cromolyn or nedocromil before exercise may prevent their symptoms. This may be especially effective for those who plan to work out outside on days when there are high pollen counts or indoors in places where levels of inhaled asthma triggers are high.

The federal government's National Asthma Education and Prevention Program has developed special guidelines for treating exercise-induced asthma, relying heavily on the pretreatment strategies. If you have asthma attacks when exercising, you should see your doctor. You and your doctor will determine the best medications for your disease. Most people with asthma find they can prevent attacks during exercise by taking 2 puffs of their beta-adrenergic asthma inhaler or two puffs of cromolyn immediately before they begin exercising. This can give 2 to 3 hours of symptom-free exercise. People who have more severe asthma or who exercise in areas where there are many inhaled asthma triggers may need to take both cromolyn and their beta-adrenergic asthma inhaler before exercise to adequately prevent an attack.

If you use the long-acting bronchodilator Serevent as part of your normal asthma care, you may find that this medication is useful for preventing exercise-induced attacks. Serevent needs to be taken at least 30 minutes before exercise, preferably 2 hours before. It usually prevents exercise-induced asthma for 4 to 6 hours. However, if you take Serevent every day, it may be less useful against exercise-induced attacks.

You should also remember to keep your inhaled beta-adrenergic inhaler handy when exercising. The National Asthma Education and Prevention Program guidelines suggest that you take 2 to 4 inhalations if you have an asthma attack when exercising. If the attack is severe, you may need to repeat the dose 5 to 10 minutes later. If this second dose still does not help, you should seek medical attention immediately.

Pretreatment Strategies to Prevent Exercise-Induced Asthma

1. Medication
Beta-adrenergic inhalers

Short-acting drugs (albuterol, bitolterol, metaproterenol, isoetharine, isoproterenol, pirbuterol, terbutaline): 2 to 4 inhalations a few minutes before exercise

Long-acting agent (salmeterol): 2 inhalations at least 30 minutes before exercise

Anti-inflammatories

Cromolyn (Intal): 2 to 4 inhalations a few minutes before exercise
Nedocromil sodium (Tilade): 2 to 4 inhalations a few minutes before exercise

2. Excercise
Warm-up exercises

15 minutes of low-level aerobics and stretching prior to exercise

Cool-down exercises

15 minutes of light exercise and stretching upon completion

Remember that inhaled steroids do not prevent exercise-induced asthma if taken right before exercise. However, if you use your inhaled steroid regularly, your asthma will be under better control and you may be less likely to have an attack whenever you exercise. Inhaled steroids and cromolyn or nedocromil do not help an attack once it has started.

Exercise-Induced Anaphylaxis

People with allergies must also be careful about exercising. Exercise-induced anaphylaxis is a rare but frightening and potentially fatal physical allergy that has been linked to eating certain foods before vigorous activity. These foods include shrimp, celery, peanuts, egg whites, almonds, and bananas. Exercise-induced anaphylaxis occurs more commonly in hot, humid weather conditions and may also be related to the severity of the exertion.

The signs of exercise-induced anaphylaxis include flushing, hives, rash, swelling of the throat, bronchospasms, and faintness. If you are at risk of anaphylaxis, you should avoid strenuous exercise immediately after eating. As always, you should carry your anaphylaxis emergency kit with you when exercising.

Regular exercise, while not a cure for asthma, increases fitness and, if undertaken appropriately, can result in less troublesome exercise-induced asthma. The inability to participate in athletic programs or recreational sports can be a handicap for children and adults alike.

Tom Dolan

Coaches and parents have been trying to pull Olympic gold medalist Tom Dolan out of the swimming pool since he was a young boy. But despite his severe asthma and allergies, this young athlete is known as one of the most dedicated and fierce competitors on the 1996 U.S. swim team.

Dolan found out he had asthma when he was about 12 years old, but by then he had already had at least 5 years of swimming under his belt. And to talk with Dolan is to know that something like asthma was not going to stop him from going after his dreams. "My doctors told me I had pretty severe asthma," Dolan says. "But this was not going to interfere with me attaining my goals."

A look at his swimming record shows that asthma hasn't held him back in the least. Dolan won the gold medal in the 400-meter individual medley at the 1996 Summer Olympic Games in Atlanta; he holds the World Record in the same event and is often referred to as the most versatile swimmer in the world. He has twice been voted U.S. Swimmer of the Year.

Dolan, a student at the University of Michigan, has severe exercise-induced asthma and allergies. The condition is a major impediment when he runs—part of the training regimen for swimmers—and appears to get worse the more he works out. "There are times that we are literally pulling him out of the pool because his asthma is acting up and he just doesn't want to stop practicing," says Dolan's college coach, Jon Urbanchek.

Dolan's condition has put some limitations on his training schedule. After a number of bouts of exercise-induced asthma, his doctors cleared him to swim but told him to slow down. They advised that he swim for shorter distances and times and to stop pushing himself at every practice. Dolan begrudgingly complied. He cut his grueling work schedule from about 12 miles of swimming a day to a little more than 4 miles.

Yet that reduced schedule didn't seem to bother him when he easily cruised to Olympic gold. Dolan uses an inhaled steroid on a regular basis and relies on an inhaled beta-adrenergic drug when he is wheezing and before exercise to reduce the chance of an exercise-induced attack.

"I don't really think about my asthma that much, except that I have to take my medications regularly," Dolan says. He has regular conversations with past Olympic swimming medalist Nancy Hogshead, who also suffers from asthma. "Nancy and I both agree that this is a condition we need to manage, but it is certainly not something that we are going to let get in the way of the things we love to do." ❏

16 / Planning Time Away from Home

ROUNDING UP THE CHILDREN, PACKING THE CAR, AND SETTING out on a family vacation is a great American tradition. Parents who have been on family vacations know that careful planning is the best way to ensure a smooth and enjoyable trip. And that is certainly the case when planning a vacation that involves a family member with asthma or allergies.

If there is one rule to asthma and allergies, it is that these conditions often flare up at the most inopportune time. Plan a vacation to the mountains to see the beautiful countryside, and you can be sure that your family member with allergies will suffer from the pollen of the wildflowers; set out on a trip to a resort or an amusement park, and chances are that your child with asthma will have an attack from running around or another trigger. Certainly not everyone with asthma or allergies has an attack while on vacation, but families with asthma and allergy sufferers know to plan for the worst. And indeed, it is by planning ahead that you can prevent these conditions from putting a damper on your time together as a family.

Vacation planning for the family with asthma or allergies presents a real challenge. Your goal in planning a trip is to minimize the chance that your family member with these conditions will suffer an attack. By properly planning ahead and sticking to the medication course pre-scribed by your doctor, you can reduce the chance that asthma or allergy attacks will spoil a vacation. Nevertheless, you also need to have a plan of action in case an asthma or allergy attack does strike while you're away from home. While no family likes to think of an attack coming in the middle of their anticipated fun, proper planning, including a strategy for handling attacks, can go a long way toward ensuring that your vacation is still a success.

The exact way you plan will depend on your specific circumstances.

You must take into account the age of your family member with asthma or allergies, the severity of the disease, your destination, and the means you are using to get there. There are some universal steps, however, that all families with asthma or allergy sufferers should follow.

The first step is to have your family member's disease under control. By following the advice in this book and consulting with your doctor about identifying and avoiding asthma and allergy triggers and using medications to prevent and reverse attacks, you or your family member should already be managing these conditions. When planning for a vacation, do not alter this treatment plan. In the excitement of an upcoming trip, controlling asthma and allergies may slip from the forefront of your mind. Avoid this temptation by being mindful that asthma and allergies that are under control are less likely to flare up while you are away from home.

To ensure that the disease is well controlled before setting out on your trip, you or your family member should visit the doctor about two months before leaving. This will allow you to make any necessary adjustments to the medication schedule and still give plenty of time to acclimate to the new schedule before your vacation. It will also give you the opportunity to address any disease symptoms that are beginning to flare up. During that visit to the doctor, ask for a disease prevention and emergency plan that you can carry with you. The plan should list all the drugs your family member is taking and which ones should be used for prevention and emergency therapy.

Planning Your Trip

Investigate asthma and allergy triggers. The climate and surroundings of your destination can play a big role in your family member's asthma or allergies. You should determine what disease triggers, such as pollen, weather changes, climate, pets, and smoke, your family member may be exposed to on your vacation. When planning time away from home, you should take the same approach to asthma and allergy triggers that you do at home. Remember that avoidance is the primary therapy. Find out what the seasonal allergens are in your destination area and whether they will be in bloom during your trip. What is the climate expected to be like? Ask your doctor about medications to prevent attacks in these new surroundings. Do the relatives you may be staying with smoke or have pets? While it may be difficult to alter your vacation plans, you must weigh the comfort and safety of your family member with asthma and allergies if you plan to stay with smokers or people who have pets.

Identify the closest hospitals. While no family wants to think they may need to go to a hospital while away on vacation, the family with asthma or allergy sufferers needs to plan for this possibility. Know the hospital closest to where you are staying in case of an emergency. This will prevent anxiety in the event that your family member has an attack and will ensure that you can get help in the quickest possible manner.

Know your mode of travel. Whether traveling by car, boat, airplane, or train, how you reach your vacation destination impacts on how you prepare for your trip. Now that all domestic flights are smoke free, planning a trip by air in the United States is easier for people with asthma or allergies. This is not the case when traveling abroad. Make sure you are seated as far from the smoking section as possible if you are on an overseas flight that allows smoking. Also be aware that even on nonsmoking flights, the dry, recirculated air on planes can play havoc with asthma and allergies. Planes are often dusty, and mold spores can build up in the ventilation systems. Ask your doctor about any special medications, such as decongestants or antihistamines, that can ease your family member's flight. Since people with asthma or allergies also frequently have sinus problems, make sure you take along plenty of fluids and chewing gum. Drinking and chewing gum can help relieve the pressure in the ears and sinuses during take-offs and landings.

Traveling by other means also requires special preparations. If your young child with asthma uses a power-driven nebulizer, make sure you get an adapter that allows the nebulizer to work off a cigarette lighter. If your nebulizer does not allow for this feature, you can rent a battery-operated device that allows for a cigarette-lighter adapter. Whether your family member with asthma uses a nebulizer or a pocket-sized inhaler with a spacer or face mask, try to time your rest stops so they occur a few minutes after administering the asthma medication. This will enable your child to play or hike at the rest stop with an adequate amount of preventive medicine already in his or her lungs.

Think ahead about your lodgings. Whether you are staying in a cabin, hotel, or tent, try to make the surroundings as free of asthma and allergy triggers as possible. Cabins and rental homes are often filled with dust and mold spores. Make sure a cleaning crew has been through the place before you arrive. When renting a cabin or home, tell the landlord about your asthma or allergies and any special cleaning you require. This is especially important if you will be the first people using the lodging for the season. Most modern hotels are very clean and have entire floors designated for nonsmokers. Check with the reservations desk and make sure you get a nonsmoking room. You may also want to bring your own nonallergenic pillow encased in a dustproof cover. While most modern hotels have nonallergenic pillows available from the housekeeping department, other accommodations may not. And even most nonallergenic pillows do not come with dust-proof covers to reduce exposure to house dust mites.

Plan your activities. While spur-of-the-moment side trips on vacations are part of what makes traveling fun, families of asthma and allergy sufferers must be prepared for these events. If you think your family may go hiking while away, take a backpack that can accommodate needed medications. If horseback riding is on the list of things to do, bring along some nonsedating antihistamines to take a few hours before the ride and also bring a fanny pack to carry inhalers and other medications. If you plan a trip to a beach, a small waterproof bag is good for carrying needed medicines.

Know how long you plan to be away. The length of your vacation will dictate how much medication you need to take along. Most asthma inhalers have enough medication when full to last a month. If you are going on an extended vacation, remember to bring an extra one. (Pack at least one backup inhaler in case one gets misplaced.) You will also want to make sure you have enough oral medications to last for your trip. If the bottle of oral medications you plan to take is not brand-new, count out how many pills are left. Families with a member who is at risk for anaphylaxis should also carry at least two anaphylaxis emergency kits. In addition:

- Have prescriptions for all medicines in case they get lost.

- Always carry medicines with you. Leaving them in the luggage in your hotel room does you no good if you have an attack at the beach or during another outdoor activity.

- If you are going to be away for a while and your child has severe disease, get the name of a specialist in that area before you leave.

Packing for Your Trip

Once you have a clear idea of where you are going, how you are getting there, where you will stay, and what your activities will be, you can begin the business of packing. This requires some special consider-

"April"

When April was seven her parents took her and her two brothers on a trip to the mountains. April's mom, Tracy, took all of April's asthma medications and thought she had planned as best as she could to take care of her daughter's asthma while away. "April hadn't had a serious asthma attack for about one year, so we thought everything would be fine," Tracy remembers.

On the second day of their trip the family went on a tour of some caverns in the area. The tour was beautiful, with the lights in the cavern illuminating the pinkish minerals in the walls. But the cold, moist, musty air turned out to be a trigger for April's asthma. "We just didn't think of that before we set out, so we didn't give April any additional medications before the tour," Tracy says. About halfway through the one-and-a-half-hour tour, April began to wheeze. Tracy gave April her inhaler, but the wheezing did not clear up as soon as usual. Tracy told one of the guides about April's asthma and that the family needed to leave. The guide escorted April's family to the nearest exit, but because they were in the middle of the cavern, it still took about 15 minutes before the family was back above ground. By then April's asthma attack had worsened.

"When we got back to the car, April was really wheezing and had all the signs of a serious asthma attack. She was gasping for breath, sucking in her chest, and coughing," Tracy says. "I wanted to give her more of her beta-adrenergic inhaler, but I knew of the dangers of overusing this drug." April's dad got the family into the car and started heading for help, but they didn't know where the closest hospital was. "We were just speeding down the highway, looking for a sign, when a policeman pulled us over for speeding," Tracy says. "Once he saw our daughter's situation, he told us to follow him and he escorted us to the nearest hospital, which was only a few minutes away. Luckily, he radioed ahead, so a doctor and nurse were waiting for us when we pulled in."

April's asthma attack had progressed to the point where she needed an injection of epinephrine to reverse the attack. When she left the hospital a few hours later, she was breathing fine but was exhausted from the excitement and attack. "It was a real learning experience for us," Tracy says. "We thought we had planned well enough for the trip by taking her medications, but we had no idea where the local hospitals were and we didn't think to give her some preventive medicine before setting out on that tour."

April and her family have been on numerous vacations since their trip to the mountains. And while April has had asthma attacks on subsequent trips, none have required a trip to the hospital. "We just plan a lot better now," says Tracy. "We know where the hospitals are and we know what activities we will be doing, so we can plan her medication schedule appropriately. April's asthma does not stop us from doing what the family wants. We have been on plenty of other trips to the mountains and she has been fine. We just know to plan our vacation with her asthma in mind."

ations for the family with asthma and allergy sufferers. By planning ahead, you can ease this part of your trip, and you can train your child with asthma and allergies how to pack when he or she takes trips without Mom and Dad. Packing for your trip requires that you think of all the medications your family member may need while away from home. Making a list of his or her conditions and medications can simplify the packing process.

1. Be sure to take enough medications with you and to refill your prescriptions before leaving home.

2. Make sure you carry at least two anaphylaxis emergency kits if someone is at risk for this serious allergic reaction. Keep one in the bag with the other medications and store the other one in a safe place like the glove compartment or a purse.

3. Pack all medications in a separate box or bag that is easy to carry. Keep this container with you at all times. If traveling by airplane, use this box or bag as a carry-on item.

4. Pack your insurance cards.

5. Keep a list of area hospitals in the bag with your medications.

6. Write out a list of all medications, with doses and times to be taken. This can be of great value if you need to visit a hospital while away.

7. Write a list of all allergies, including insects, drugs, foods, etc. This list can help doctors who do not know your disease history.

8. Bring two summaries of your family member's asthma or allergy history. Include ideal and trouble peak flow readings, all medications used, and a history of serious attacks. Keep one list in the medication bag and put the other in a wallet or purse.

9. Be sure to take enough nebulizer supplies if one is used. Pack the compressor and supplies in a separate bag. Be sure the battery is charged if there is one for the nebulizer, or take along a cigarette lighter adapter cord. Make sure you pack all cords, tubing, and other attachments.

10. Make sure the affected family member wears a Medic Alert bracelet or necklace listing his or her asthma and allergies.

11. Get a set of prescriptions in case you lose medications or need a refill.

When Your Child Vacations Without You

Whether to send your child off on a vacation without you can be a decision filled with anxiety. Will he or she continue to take medications appropriately? What if he or she has an asthma attack? Who will be supervising, and do they understand how to manage and treat asthma and allergies? Whether you are deciding to send your child on a vacation with relatives or friends or are considering a summer camp, these are the questions you will need to answer.

The first thing to do to prepare your child for a vacation without you is to make sure he or she understands the disease and how to manage it. Children with asthma and allergies are quite adept at managing their own condition. With proper training, they can learn to recognize the signs of an impending attack better than anyone else. As parents, you need to make sure your child is comfortable managing his or her own disease. Make sure your child knows what medications to use regularly and which to use in case of an emergency. It is very important that he or she knows not to overuse the beta-adrenergic inhaler when wheezing. Instruct your child on how much of this medication can be used in one day and make it clear that if breathing is still difficult, he or she should seek other help. Teach your child how to monitor his or her asthma with a peak flow meter. Educate your child in the use of an anaphylaxis emergency kit if this allergic reaction is a possibility.

The American Lung Association recommends that before sending your child on a vacation, you:

- Make sure your child knows his or her asthma triggers.

- Make sure he or she can recognize the beginnings of an attack and how to respond.

- Provide a list of your child's allergies to the supervisor on the trip.

- Also include a history and severity of your child's asthma, including recent hospital visits.

- Provide a list of your child's medications, including type, dose, and times taken.

- Provide prescriptions for drug renewals.

Once your child knows about his or her disease and how to manage it, make sure that all medications and other asthma and allergy tools are packed. It is your job to determine that your child takes all needed medications, information sheets, and insurance cards on the trip. By following these steps, you can reduce the chance that your child will suffer an attack while away and make it a little easier for yourself to sleep at night until your child returns home.

If you plan to send your child with asthma to a summer camp, there are other things you should do to make his or her vacation enjoyable. If you are sending your child to an asthma camp, the American Lung Association recommends you make sure that the camp furnishes equipment to measure your child's pulmonary function. The asthma camp also should provide a sufficient supply of routine asthma medications and equipment, including bronchodilators, corticosteroids, nebulizers, and peak flow meters. (When sending your child to a regular summer camp, it is your responsibility to provide your child with a peak flow meter and asthma medications.) You should make sure that any summer camp your child is attending:

- has an adequate camper-to-nurse ratio

- has procedures to treat asthma attacks

- requires that at least one nurse skilled in asthma management is in the infirmary at all times

- has physician and urgent care readily available

It is also a good idea to send a letter to the camp supervisor or vacation chaperone giving details of your child's asthma and allergies. If possible, try to meet with them in person or have a phone conversation before your child leaves for camp. Be sure to inform the supervisor, camp counselor, or chaperone about your child's disease and his or her asthma and allergy triggers. Indicate all medications that your child uses and what to do in case of an emergency. On page 197 is a sample letter you can use when sending your child off on a vacation.

Asthma Camps

To help educate children about asthma while also giving them the opportunity to get out in nature, the American Lung Association and other organizations sponsor children's asthma camps. Asthma camps are built on the principle that children can learn to control their own disease. Throughout the one- to two-week programs, children learn the specifics of asthma management, including how to recognize their triggers and how to use an asthma inhaler correctly.

INFORMATION FOR CAMP SUPERVISORS OR VACATION CHAPERONES

My child, _____, has asthma. The condition should not prevent him/her from taking part in usual activities. However, there are occasions when his/her asthma may flare up. During an asthma flare-up, he/she should not go out in the cold or participate in strenuous physical activity. My child understands his/her disease and how to manage it. He/she knows when to use an inhaler and other asthma medications. Please listen to my child if he/she says it is time for an asthma medication, or in the event that he/she decides not to participate in an activity because of asthma. My child knows best how his/her disease works.

_____ must take the following medications at the hours noted to control his/her condition (check those that apply):

___ theophylline, _____ mg, at _____.

___ cromolyn, _____ puffs, at _____.

___ inhaled steroids, _____ puffs, at _____.

___ inhaled beta-adrenergics, _____ puffs, at _____.

___ He/she also uses an inhaler before sports and if wheezing during physical activity.

Please let me know if I can provide you with more information regarding my child's condition or medications. Attached you will find the emergency asthma care plan developed by my child's doctor in case of an emergency.

If you have any questions, please call me at home, _____, or at work, _____.

If you can't reach me, please call _____, who is apprised of my child's condition, or our physician, Dr. _____, at _____.

Sincerely,

_____

Attending asthma camp can be an excellent way for your child to learn about asthma. A study of 90 children with asthma between the ages of 6 and 12 who attended a summer camp program found that the children were more knowledgeable and better able to control their disease after the experience. While only about half the children used a spacer with the asthma inhaler upon starting the camp, 92 percent used one at the end of the program and 86 percent continued using a spacer 6 months after the camp ended. The use of peak flow meters also increased among the children. About half used the meters when they started camp, with 95 percent measuring their own peak flow after camp training and 88 percent continuing to do so 6 months later. The researchers concluded that the training the children received in the camp was the likely reason that they had far fewer hospital visits and school absences after the program than they had before going to camp.

Asthma camps are not just for teaching youngsters how to control their disease. They are filled with the same activities typical of other summer camps, such as craft classes, nature hikes, swimming, and boating. Yet the activities are made safe for children with asthma, since most of the camps have a full staff of respiratory care specialists, nurses, and doctors.

A VACATION CHECKLIST

❑ Consult with doctor to adjust medication schedule if necessary.

❑ Continue with preventive medication plan.

❑ Refill all prescriptions.

❑ Get extra prescription for refills while away in the event medications are lost.

❑ Obtain extra anaphylaxis emergency kit.

❑ Make list of asthma and allergy triggers, and of medications and their doses and times.

❑ Make two lists of asthma emergency plan with best and worst peak flow readings and history of serious attacks.

❑ Buy new battery or cigarette-lighter adapter cord for nebulizer.

❑ Get backpack and fanny pack to store medications when hiking or away from the car or lodging.

❑ Reserve nonsmoking airplane seats and hotel rooms.

❑ Call ahead to make sure cleaning crew has prepared cabin.

❑ Locate and list the hospitals nearest to where you are traveling.

❑ Take insurance cards.

❑ Bring a nonallergenic pillow encased in a dustproof cover.

At an asthma camp children can learn to manage their disease themselves in an atmosphere of support and with a staff that understands asthma care. They develop a sense of independence by managing their disease alone and away from their parents. And there is no stigma at the camps because children see one another using inhalers and other asthma medications and tools. If you are interested in sending your child with asthma to an asthma summer camp, contact your local chapter of the American Lung Association or see the directory of camps at the end of this book.

17 / The Costs of Asthma and Allergies

ASTHMA AND ALLERGIES ARE CHRONIC DISEASES ASSOCIATED with enormous costs. It is estimated that the total cost of asthma care is about $12.6 billion a year, including medical care, lost wages from missing work, and lost productivity. Treating allergies, particularly allergic rhinitis, totals about $2 billion a year for physician visits, diagnostic tests, medications, and immunotherapy. People with allergies rack up 8.4 million physician visits a year, costing some $225 million. Allergies also cost society an additional $3.4 million in lost wages and $639 million in lost productivity.

Families bear the brunt of these costs. Paying for medications, doctor visits, hospital stays, and emergency room treatment can take a big bite out of the family budget. These expenses, while substantial, represent only part of the bill associated with asthma and allergies. The families of people with asthma and allergies can also face financial strains when parents must miss work to care for a child who is having an asthma attack or when a spouse is so debilitated by allergies that he or she cannot go about the daily routine.

Insurance plans can help cover many of the medical costs associated with asthma and allergies, but even with the best of coverage, families must face a significant financial liability. Traditional insurance plans often do not begin paying for care until a yearly deductible is met, and even after a family pays that deductible, significant co-payments can help to empty the wallet. Health maintenance plans allow patients to visit doctors at a fraction of the cost incurred when paying out of pocket. Many HMOs also offer reduced prices or minimal co-payments for prescription drugs; this can add up to significant savings with diseases like asthma and allergies, which require the regular, long-term use of costly medications. But the cost savings associated with HMOs do not come without a sacrifice. Some HMOs restrict patients from seeing specialists, mandating instead that people with asthma and allergies have their conditions treated by general practitioners or primary-care doctors. While this type of approach may be fine for people with mild to moderate asthma and allergies or those whose asthma is already under control, some people with difficult-to-control asthma may need to see a specialist who can properly diagnose the condition and start them on a tailor-made maintenance plan.

The cheapest and most effective way to treat asthma and allergies is by properly controlling them. By following the advice in this book, you can prevent and reduce the severity and frequency of many attacks. Properly controlled asthma and allergies mean fewer attacks, fewer visits to doctors and hospitals, less time missed from work or school, and a better quality of life. Many insurers are beginning to realize that by promoting better control of asthma and allergies, they can save money in the long run by reducing costly hospital and doctor visits. In an effort to promote this type of care, some companies have begun asthma self-management programs, in which people with asthma can learn about their disease and how to manage it.

This chapter begins with a look at some of the options for paying for asthma and allergy care, from HMOs to traditional insurance plans. Next comes a discussion of some new strategies for managing these diseases that can reduce costs and result in better care, and in conclusion, some tips to reduce your family's financial burden of paying for asthma and allergies.

HMOs vs. Traditional Insurance

By now most Americans have heard of HMOs, which have grown to cover an increasingly large portion of the health insurance market. Simply put, these plans provide insurance for a fixed cost, covering everything from doctor visits and medications to hospital stays and emergency treatment. The typical plan allows members to visit their doctor or an emergency room for a nominal co-payment, in the range of $2 to $25 per visit. Many plans also cover prescription medications, with members having to pay only $5 to $10 per prescription. This can represent a significant savings for people with asthma and allergies, many of whom must take medications on a daily basis. Without this coverage, the cost of an asthma inhaler, for instance, can range from $30 to $90, with each inhaler holding enough medication for about one month.

But HMOs can have a downside. Many plans limit whether

members can see a specialist. Typically, a person in an HMO must first see a primary-care doctor for evaluation. This is called the gatekeeper concept, since the primary-care doctor is seen as the gateway a person must pass through before seeing a specialist. If the primary-care doctor feels the condition is serious enough to warrant seeing a specialist, he or she makes a referral, which is covered in the same manner as the initial visit to the generalist. However, primary-care doctors in many HMOs receive financial incentives to restrict the number of referrals they make. Consequently, you may find your primary-care doctor reluctant to refer you to an asthma specialist. If you are covered by an HMO and do not think your asthma is under good control and have not seen an asthma specialist, ask your primary-care doctor to refer you. Depending on your doctor and the HMO, you may have to insist that your disease be initially treated by an asthma specialist.

By the same token, many people with mild to moderate asthma can get excellent care from generalist physicians, such as internists or family physicians. If you are under the care of a generalist and you think your asthma may not be under good control, there are some signs to look for:

- You should be able to sleep through the night without waking because of your asthma.

- You should be able to be fully active and take part in the activities you want to.

- You should be able to get through a cold or flu without significant asthma symptoms.

If you do not fit all these criteria, it may be time for you to see a specialist. Talk to your generalist and explain that you are having trouble with your asthma.

Some HMOs have begun to make access to an asthma specialist easier, while others have started to implement programs to teach people with asthma about their disease and how to manage it. In fact, some HMOs allow people with asthma to see a specialist after first consulting with their generalist. Many people in HMOs receive health insurance from their employer and thus have little or no choice of plan. Some employers, however, offer a choice between different types of insurance coverage and even among different HMOs. If you are in the market for an HMO, there are some things you can look for when deciding whether a particular HMO is right for you.

First, determine if the HMO you are looking into has a gatekeeper system, and if it does, try to determine how difficult it will be for you to see an asthma specialist. Some plans contract with individual doctors, meaning you may have to go see a primary-care specialist before making a separate trip to a different part of town to see a specialist. Other plans contract with groups of doctors, and you may find that the office in which your primary-care doctor works also employs an asthma specialist.

Next, find out how much you have to co-pay for each prescription drug and if the plan limits the amount or type of drugs your doctor can prescribe. While some plans allow doctors to prescribe whatever drug is deemed appropriate, others mandate that a generic drug or medication from a list of drugs approved by the HMO be used. If this is the case, you'll want to find out if the drugs your doctor can prescribe are best for your disease.

You will also want to find out whether the HMO offers an asthma management program. These programs can be an excellent tool for educating people about asthma, how to control it, and what triggers can cause an attack.

Tips for Picking an HMO

- Check to see if the plan has a gatekeeper system.

- Determine whether an asthma specialist is in the same office as your primary-care doctor.

- Ask whether there are limitations or caps on emergency room treatment.

- Find out about restrictions on the medications your doctor can prescribe.

- Check what the prescription drug co-payment is.

- Find out if there are limits on how much asthma or allergy medication you can get at any one time.

- Determine whether the HMO will pay for non-drug-related asthma costs, such as the purchase of a nebulizer, peak flow meter, or other asthma care necessities.

- Ask whether the HMO has an asthma management or education program.

Selecting an HMO can be a difficult decision, but if you follow these steps, you can pick a plan that offers high-quality asthma management while significantly reducing the cost of your regular prescriptions and emergency treatment. A properly run HMO can provide you with good care at a significant cost savings over traditional insurance.

If HMOs offer inexpensive care with some restrictions, traditional insurance is their antithesis. People enrolled in traditional insurance plans can see any doctor they wish whenever they want, but for the most part they must pay for it. These plans typically impose a yearly deductible, which is a specified amount of money the insured must pay for health care before the plan starts covering any costs. These deductibles can range from a few hundred dollars to a few thousand. Even after the yearly deductible is met, the out-of-pocket expenses do not stop. Most traditional insurance plans do not cover all expenses but rather a fixed percentage of costs after the deductible. While this percentage varies, 80 percent is typical.

Remember that asthma is a disease that costs far more to maintain when it is poorly controlled. Poorly controlled asthma results in increased doctor and hospital visits and the possibility of costly emergency treatment. Asthma also costs more to control in the beginning phases of developing a treatment plan. Once a treatment plan is developed and the disease is under control, you will find that the costs associated with asthma will fall.

This means that families with asthma and allergy sufferers can spend a lot of their own money on medical costs. One study of 36 families in which a child had asthma illustrates how expensive this care can be. The families were enrolled in traditional insurance plans yet spent an average of $1,987.19 a year on asthma care, or more than 6 percent of their total yearly income, including $358 on doctor fees, $233 on medications, and $204 on hospital costs. Another study found that the average yearly cost per person with asthma is about $640 in 1990 dollars.

If you are trying to decide between an HMO and a traditional insurance plan, you should try to determine which plan offers the best possible care for the least amount of money. Calculate how much asthma medication, how many emergency room visits, and how many doctor visits you or your family member has had in the last year and try to project what a year's worth of care would cost in either plan. Then consider the intangible factors. If the doctor you have been seeing for years is not a part of the HMO your employer is offering, you must ask yourself whether saving a few dollars is worth changing doctors.

Remember that as the face of the health insurance industry changes there are ever more options available. For instance, a point-of-service plan is an option that provides HMO-like care but allows members to see nonmember physicians at an extra charge. This type of plan may be an option for those who want the flexibility of seeing nonmember specialists. The important thing to remember is to investigate all the health insurance options available to you and your family.

Changing the Insurance Industry

Whether your family is covered by an HMO, a traditional insurance policy, or a government plan such as Medicaid, you want to make sure you get the best asthma care available. To help ensure that insurers provide high-quality asthma care, the federal government's National Asthma Education and Prevention Program has released a list of recommendations it thinks insurers should follow regarding asthma care. While these guidelines are meant for insurance executives and policy makers, families with asthma should also know about them. Some of the recommendations offer hints about what to look for in an insurance policy.

The National Asthma Education and Prevention Program recommends that insurers:

- *Make asthma care affordable and accessible by keeping out-of-pocket expenses to a minimum.* Middle-class families should have to pay no more than 5 percent of their total annual income on asthma care, while families below the poverty level in their state should pay nothing for care.

- *Eliminate barriers to coverage, such as limitations on insurance coverage for preexisting conditions.* The program recommends that people with asthma be able to switch insurance policies without the fear of not being accepted by the new company because of their condition.

- *Eliminate deductibles and limit the amount of co-payment for inpatient and emergency asthma care.* Because asthma emergency care can be a matter of life and death, the program urges that health insurance reform legislation be enacted to ensure that finances will not deter people from seeking care. It also recommends that people with asthma be required to go for periodic checkups.

- *Eliminate restrictive controls on drug benefits.* Since many insurance plans limit covering prescriptions to 30-day supplies, the program recommends that people with asthma be exempt from this policy.

- *Ensure coverage of durable medical equipment with a lengthy authorization period.* This would allow families with children who have asthma to purchase nebulizers and other asthma goods without having to wait for an insurance company to approve the purchase in advance.

- *Offer free or low-cost formal asthma education programs through health plans.* These services, which now are offered on a voluntary basis by only a minority of plans, can improve asthma maintenance and cut costs by reducing visits to the emergency room.

- *Maintain uninterrupted health coverage for all people with asthma who are involved in workers' compensation claims throughout the duration of the proceedings.* This would ensure that people with asthma continue to have their disease controlled while awaiting the outcome of any unemployment claims.

Asthma Education Programs

Asthma is a disease that is best managed through partnerships. By involving people with asthma in the control, maintenance, and care of their condition, doctors believe that the disease can be better controlled and less expensive. The cost savings are apparent because people with asthma who are well educated about their disease have fewer attacks requiring expensive emergency treatment.

In recent years asthma education programs have been developed to teach people with asthma about their disease and how to control it so they can reduce the frequency and severity of attacks. Through these programs, people with asthma learn to monitor their breathing with a peak flow meter, use an inhaler correctly, recognize the signs of an impending asthma attack, and identify and avoid common asthma triggers and promoters. Numerous studies have shown that asthma education programs are an effective way to reduce hospitalizations for asthma, reduce the number of attacks, and save money.

The program can be inexpensive to operate. One study of 267 adults with asthma found that an asthma education program could be conducted for about $28 per person. Another study found that a one-year program given to 241 adults with asthma reduced emergency room visits from 39 per 100 patients to 16. The program cost $82 per person to run but saved $628 per person in reduced hospital charges.

These types of studies indicate how effective education can be at controlling asthma and reducing the costs of care. If you are interested in taking part in an asthma education program, call your insurance company's benefits office or your local hospitals and medical facilities. Many of these facilities conduct similar programs, most of which are free of charge. You can also get a list of programs in your area by contacting the National Asthma Education and Prevention Program (listed in the Asthma and Allergy Resources at the end of this book).

Watching Your Wallet

By now you can appreciate the need to properly control your asthma and allergies. Asthma and allergies are chronic diseases that can flare up at almost any time. An uncontrolled disease results in frequent attacks and can interfere with the ability to lead a normal, constructive life. By controlling your disease, you can lead a normal life and know what to do when a rare attack does strike. There is a financial reason to control your asthma and allergies as well. People with properly controlled conditions spend far less money on their diseases. They do not have to visit the hospital and doctors' offices as often, thus cutting down on expensive emergency care.

If you have asthma or allergies, the best way to reduce your health care bill is by following the steps in this book on how to best control your disease. You may find that in the initial phase your bill for asthma care actually increases because of visits to the doctor and new medications and devices you may be required to use. You will save money in the long run, however, when your asthma or allergies do not flare up as often. You will make fewer visits to the emergency room, and you will miss less time from school or work.

While you strive for the best possible ways to control your disease, there are some other steps you can take to trim costs. Try following these tips to get the best asthma care possible for the least money:

- *Examine your drug benefits.* If everything else is equal, choose an insurance plan that has low co-payments for prescription drugs, as long as there are no restrictions on what types of drugs your doctor can prescribe. You should also call your insurance company to see if it has a prescription-by-mail program. These programs offer people the opportunity to purchase their regularly used prescriptions through the mail at a substantial cost savings. Insurance plans that offer low co-payments for prescription drugs or have a mail-order program can save you significant money on your medication costs.

- *Shop around.* The prices of nebulizers and other asthma equipment can vary greatly from one pharmacy or medical supply store to the next. Ask your doctor which models are best for your child with asthma and call a few stores for prices.

- *Reuse your mouthpiece.* You may be able to buy new canisters of asthma medications without having to purchase the entire inhaler. These refills may be cheaper than buying the inhaler and mouthpiece together. Remember to carefully clean your mouthpiece with soap and water and allow it to dry if you plan to reuse it. Check with your pharmacy to see if it sells canister refills—you can save some money and protect the environment by using less plastic.

- *Try to get it free.* Spacers and peak flow meters are sometimes given out free of charge as promotions by pharmaceutical companies or asthma education programs. Call the maker of the asthma medication you are using or your local hospital's or insurance company's asthma education program to see if either has this program.

- *Educate yourself.* Free asthma education programs can be an excellent way to learn about your disease while also saving money managing it. Many of these courses offer reduced rates on certain prescriptions and other asthma essentials. It can't hurt to attend a free course, and you just might learn something.

By following these tips, you will find that saving money is a welcome benefit of properly controlled asthma or allergies. Maybe you will want to use some of those extra dollars to take a trip and get outdoors now that your asthma or allergies will not be stopping you anymore.

DIRECTORY OF ASTHMA CAMPS

Many of these camps are sponsored by the American Lung Association. Please call individual camps for information on dates and facilities available.

ALABAMA
Montgomery
CAMP WHEEZEAWAY
1425B I-85 Parkway
Montgomery, AL 36106
334-277-7195

ALASKA
Anchorage
CHAMP CAMP
1057 W. Fireweed Lane, #201
Anchorage, AK 99503-1736
907-276-5864

ARIZONA
Phoenix
CAMP NOT-A-WHEEZE
102 W. McDowell Road
Phoenix, AZ 85003
602-258-7505

ARKANSAS
Little Rock
ASTHMA CAMP
211 Natural Resources Drive
Little Rock, AR 72205-1539
501-224-5864

CALIFORNIA
Chico
CAMP SUPERSTUFF
1108 N. Sheridan Avenue, Suite B
Chico, CA 95926
916-345-5864

Daly City
CAMP SUPERSTUFF
2171 Junipero Serra Boulevard, #720
Daly City, CA 94014-1999
415-994-5864

Fresno
CAMP SIERRA
4948 N. Arthur
Fresno, CA 93705
209-266-5864

Long Beach
ALA of Los Angeles County/CSULB
ASTHMA CAMP
CSU, Long Beach, Department
of Physical Education
1250 Bell Flower Boulevard
Long Beach, CA 90840
562-985-7969

Los Angeles
BARLOW RESPIRATORY
HOSPITAL
ALA of Los Angeles County
5858 Wilshire Boulevard., Ste. 300
Los Angeles, CA 90036
213-935-5864

Oakland
BREATHE EASY DAY CAMP
295 27th Street
Oakland, CA 94612
510-893-5474

Pleasant Hill
CHAMP CAMP AND ASTHMA
DAY CAMP
105 Astrid Drive
Pleasant Hill, CA 94523
510-935-0472

San Diego
SCAMP CAMP
2750 Fourth Avenue
San Diego, CA 92103
619-297-3901

San Jose
CAMP SUPERSTUFF
1469 Park Avenue
San Jose, CA 95126
408-998-5864

Santa Ana
SCAMP CAMP
1570 E. 17th Street
Santa Ana, CA 92705
714-835-5864

Santa Barbara
CAMP WHEEZ
1510 San Andres Street
Santa Barbara, CA 93101

Santa Rosa

ASTHMA EDUCATION
DAY CAMP
P.O. Box 1482
Santa Rosa, CA 95402
707-527-5864

COLORADO

Denver

CHAMP CAMP
1600 Race Street
Denver, CO 80206
303-388-4327

CONNECTICUT

East Hartford

CAMP TREASURE CHEST
45 Ash Street
East Hartford, CT 06108
203-289-5401

DELAWARE

Wilmington

ASTHMA CAMP
1021 Gilpin Avenue, #202
Wilmington, DE 19806-3280
302-655-7258

DISTRICT of COLUMBIA

Washington

CAMP HAPPY LUNGS
475 H Street NW
Washington, DC 20001
202-682-5864

FLORIDA

Jacksonville

SUNSHINE STATION
P.O. Box 8127
Jacksonville, FL 32239
904-743-2933

GEORGIA

Atlanta

THE RITE ASTHMA CAMP
1001 Johnson Ferry Road
Atlanta, GA 30342
404-250-2654

Columbus

SUPERSTUFF ASTHMA
DAY CAMP
4570 Reese Road
Columbus, GA 31907
706-569-1098

Smyrna

CAMP BREATHE EASY
2452 Spring Road
Smyrna, GA 30080
770-434-5864, ext. 214

HAWAII

Honolulu

ASTHMA CAMP
245 N. Kukui Street, #100
Honolulu, HI 96817
808-537-5966

ILLINOIS

Chicago

CAMP ACTION
1440 W. Washington Boulevard
Chicago, IL 60607-1878
312-243-2000

Springfield

CAMP SUPERKIDS
1 Christmas Seal Drive
P.O. Box 2576
Springfield, IL 62708
217-528-3441

INDIANA

Indianapolis

CAMP SUPERKIDS
9410 Priority Way W.
Indianapolis, IN 46240
317-573-3900

South Bend

CAMP SUPERKIDS
RESIDENT CAMP
319 S. Main Street
South Bend, IN 46601
219-287-2321

IOWA

West Des Moines

CAMP SUPERKIDS
1025 Ashworth Road, #410
West Des Moines, IA 50265
515-224-0800

KANSAS

Topeka

CAMP SUPERBREATHERS
4300 Drury Lane
Topeka, KS 66604
913-272-9290

KENTUCKY

Louisville

CAMP SUPERKIDS
P.O. Box 9067
Louisville, KY 40209-0067

LOUISIANA

Opelousas

CAMP AZZIE
Prather Pediatric Asthma
& Allergy Center
3400 Highway 182 South
Opelousas, LA 70570
318-948-9606

MAINE

Augusta

CAMP OPPORTUNITY
122 State Street
Augusta, ME 04330
207-622-6394

MARYLAND

Hagerstown

CAMP BREATHE EASY
251 E. Antietam Street
Hagerstown, MD 21740
301-790-8192

Laytonsville

CAMP FRIENDSHIP
Laytonsville, MD 20760
800-492-7527 or 410-560-2120

MASSACHUSETTS

Brighton

CAMP CHEST NUT
1505 Commonwealth Avenue
Brighton, MA 02135
617-787-5864

Walpole

ASTHMA CAMP
25 Spring Street
Walpole, MA 02081
508-668-6729

MICHIGAN

Hudson

CAMP MICHI-MAC
607 Grove Street
Hudson, MI 49247
517-448-8543

Southfield

CAMP SUN DEER
18860 W. Ten Mile Road
Southfield, MI 48075
810-559-5100

MINNESOTA

Duluth

CAMP WE NO WHEEZE NORTH
424 W. Superior Street, #203
Duluth, MN 55802
218-726-4721

LITCHFIELD

*CAMP WE-NO-WHEEZE
CENTRAL*
110 N. Sibley Avenue
Litchfield, MN 55355
800-693-5864

Minneapolis

*CAMP SUPERTOTS/CAMP
SUPERTEENS/CAMP SUPERKIDS*
4220 Old Shakopee Road, #101
Minneapolis, MN 55437-2974
612-885-0338

Saint Paul

CAMP WE-NO-WHEEZE NORTH
490 Concordia Avenue
Saint Paul, MN 55103-2441
612-227-8014

Winona

CAMP WE-NO-WHEEZE
855 Mankato Avenue
P.O. Box 5600
Winona, MN 55987-0600
507-457-4332

MISSOURI

Saint Louis

CAMP SUPERKIDS
1118 Hampton Avenue
Saint Louis, MO 63139-3196
314-645-5505

GRACE HILL WELLNESS
INITIATIVE
2600 Hadley Street
Saint Louis, MO 63106
314-340-3206

MONTANA
Helena

CAMP HUFF 'N PUFF
825 Helena Avenue
Helena, MT 59601
406-442-6556

NEBRASKA
Omaha

CAMP SUPERKIDS
7101 Newport Avenue, #303
Omaha, NE 68152
402-572-3030

NEVADA
Las Vegas

CAMP SUPERKIDS
P.O. Box 44137
Las Vegas, NV 89116
702-431-6333

Reno

CHAMP CAMP
6119 Ridgeview Court, #100
Reno, NV 89509
702-829-5864

NEW HAMPSHIRE
Manchester

CAMP SUPER KIDS
456 Beech Street
P.O. Box 1014
Manchester, NH 03105
603-669-2411

NEW JERSEY
Union

CAMP SUPERKIDS
1600 Route 22 East
Union, NJ 07083-3407
908-687-9340

NEW MEXICO
Albuquerque

ASTHMA CAMP
216 Truman NE
Albuquerque, NM 87108
505-265-0732

NEW YORK
Albany

SUPERKIDS ASTHMA CAMP
8 Mountainview Avenue
Albany, NY 12205
518-459-4197

Utica

CAMP SUPERKIDS
311 Turner Street, #415
Utica, NY 13501
317-735-9225

NORTH CAROLINA
Asheville

MOUNTAIN AIR
390 S. French Broad
Asheville, NC 28801
704-254-5366

Charlotte

CAMP AIR CARE
5315 Greenbrook Drive
Charlotte, NC 28205-6521
704-537-5776

Greenville

CAMP SEA BREATHE
P.O. Box 1407
Greenville, NC 27835-1407
800-849-5949

Raleigh

CAMP CHALLENGE
3901 Barrett Drive, #313
Raleigh, NC 27609
919-782-2888

NORTH DAKOTA
Bismarck

DAKOTA SUPERKIDS
ASTHMA CAMP
P.O. Box 5004
Bismarck, ND 58502-5004
701-223-5613

OHIO
Cincinnati

CAMP SUPERKIDS
11113 Kenwood Road
Cincinnati, OH 45242
513-985-3990

Dayton

CAMP SUPERKIDS
7560 McEwen Road
Dayton, OH 45459
513-291-0451

Norwalk

CAMP SUPERKIDS AT
CAMP TIMBERLANE
226 State Route 61 E
Norwalk, OH 44857
419-663-5864

Toledo

CAMP SUPERKIDS
4759 Violet Road
Toledo, OH 43623
419-471-0024

OKLAHOMA

Tulsa

ASTHMA CAMP
2805 E. Skelly Drive, #806
Tulsa, OK 74105
918-747-3441

OREGON

Portland

CAMP CHRISTMAS SEAL
9320 SW Barbur Boulevard, #140
Portland, OR 97219-5481
503-246-1997

PENNSYLVANIA

Bethlehem

CAMP WHEEZE-AWAY
2121 Cityline Road
Bethlehem, PA 18017-2100
610-867-4100

Cranberry Township

CAMP BREATHE E-Z
Cranberry Professional Park
201 Smith Drive
Cranberry Township, PA 16066
800-220-1990 or 772-1750

East Stroudsburg

UPWARD BOUND
ASTHMA CAMP
206 E. Brown Street
East Stroudsburg, PA 18301
717-476-3522

Erie

CAMP SUPERTEEN/CAMP
SUPERSTUFF
352 W. Eighth Street
Erie, PA 16502
814-454-0109 or 800-352-0917

Harrisburg

CAMP BREATHE EASY
6041 Linglestown Road
Harrisburg, PA 17112-1208
717-541-5864

Plymouth Meeting

CAMP SUPERSTUFF
525 Plymouth Road, #315
Plymouth Meeting, PA 19462
610-941-9595

State College

CAMP SUPERKIDS
205 E. Beaver Avenue, #203
State College, PA 16801-4903
814-234-8037

Warrendale

CAMP HUFF 'N PUFF
P.O. Box 100
Warrendale, PA 15086
412-772-1750 or 800-220-1990

Williamsport

CAMP PUFF 'N' STUFF
1201 Grampian Boulevard, #1C
Williamsport, PA 17701-1900
717-326-8270

SOUTH CAROLINA

Charleston

CAMP PUFF 'N STUFF
1941 Savage Road, #200A
Charleston, SC 29407
803-556-8451

SOUTH DAKOTA

Sioux Falls

McKENNAN AIRWAY CARE
"MAC" CAMP
800 E. 21st Street
Sioux Falls, SD 57117-5045
800-331-2273 or 800-223-1558

TENNESSEE

Chattanooga

CAMP OCOEE
301 W. Sixth Street
Chattanooga, TN 37402
615-265-0455

TEXAS
Dallas
CAMP JEFFREY GREEN
7616 LBJ Freeway, #100
Dallas, TX 75251
972-239-5864

Fort Worth
CAMP BRONCHO
6420 Southwest Boulevard, #113
Fort Worth, TX 76109-9166
817-732-6336

Houston
CAMP WENOWHEEZE
P.O. Box 301093
Houston, TX 77230-1093
713-770-3392

San Antonio
CAMP BRONCHO
4502 Centerview Drive, #116
San Antonio, TX 78228
210-734-5864

Tyler
TEXAS ASTHMA CAMP
P.O. Box 2003
Tyler, TX 75710
903-877-7075

UTAH
Salt Lake City
CAMP WYATT
1930 S. 1100 East
Salt Lake City, UT 84106
801-484-4456

VERMONT
South Burlington
ASTHMA CAMP
30 Farrell Street
South Burlington, VT 05403
802-863-6817

VIRGINIA
Radford
*CAMP WHEEZER ASTHMA
DAY CAMP OF THE
NEW RIVER VALLEY*
700 Randolph Street
Radford, VA 24141-2430
540-731-2645

Richmond
CAMP SUPERKIDS
311 S. Boulevard
Richmond, VA 23221-0065
804-355-3295 or 800-345-LUNG

WASHINGTON
Tacoma
*CAMP BREATHE EASY/CAMP
CHAMP/ASTHMA CAMP AT
CAMP SEALTH*
223 Tacoma Avenue South
Tacoma, WA 98402-2513
253-272-8777

WEST VIRGINIA
Charleston
CAMP CATCH YOUR BREATH
415 Dickinson Street
Charleston, WV 25301
304-342-6600

WISCONSIN
Brookfield
*CAMP WIKIDAS (WISCONSIN
KIDS WITH ASTHMA)*
150 S. Sunnyslope Road, #105
Brookfield, WI 53005
414-782-7833

Green Bay
ASTHMA CAMP
835 S. Van Buren
Green Bay, WI 54307-3008
414-431-3042

CANADA
Halifax, Nova Scotia
CAMP TIDNISH
3670 Kemf Road
Halifax, Nova Scotia B3K 4X8
902-429-3420

ASTHMA AND ALLERGY RESOURCES

The American Lung Association and Affiliated Associations

National Office
American Lung Association
1740 Broadway
New York, NY 10019-4374
212-315-8700
http://www.lungusa.org
America Online Keyword: ALA

Government Relations Office
American Lung Association/American
Thoracic Society Washington Office
1726 M Street NW, Suite 902
Washington, DC 20036-4502
202-785-3355

The American Lung Association offers a wealth of asthma information online, from the latest asthma news to chat groups and message boards. By dialing 1-800-LUNG-USA from anywhere in the country, you are routed automatically to your local American Lung Association.

ALABAMA

ALA of Alabama
900 S. 18th Street
Birmingham, AL 35205
205-933-8821

ALASKA

ALA of Alaska
1057 W. Fireweed Lane, Suite 201
Anchorage, AK 99503-1736
907-276-5864

ARIZONA

ALA of Arizona
102 W. McDowell Road
Phoenix, AZ 85003-1299
602-258-7505

ARKANSAS

ALA of Arkansas
211 Natural Resources Drive
Little Rock, AR 72205-1539
501-224-5864

CALIFORNIA

ALA of California
424 Pendleton Way
Oakland, CA 94621-2189
510-638-5864

ALA of Alameda County
295 27th Street
Oakland, CA 94612-3894
510-893-5474

ALA of Central California
4948 N. Arthur
Fresno, CA 93705
209-222-4800

ALA of the Central Coast
174 Carmelito Avenue
Monterey, CA 93940
408-373-7306

ALA of Contra Costa–Solano
105 Astrid Drive
Pleasant Hill, CA 94523-4399
510-935-0472

ALA of the Inland Counties
441 Mac Kay Drive
San Bernardino, CA 92408-3230
909-884-5864

ALA of Los Angeles County
5858 Wilshire Boulevard, Suite 300
Los Angeles, CA 90036-0926
213-935-5864

ALA of Orange County
1570 E. 17th Street
Santa Ana, CA 92705
714-835-5864

ALA of the Redwood Empire
1301 Farmers Lane, Suite 303
Santa Rosa, CA 95405
707-527-5864

ALA of Sacramento–Emigrant Trails
909 12th Street
Sacramento, CA 95814-2997
916-444-5864

ALA of San Diego & Imperial Counties
2750 Fourth Avenue
San Diego, CA 92103
619-297-3901

ALA of San Francisco & San Mateo Counties
2171 Junipero Serra Boulevard, Suite 720
Daly City, CA 94014-1980
415-994-5864

ALA of Santa Barbara County
1510 San Andres Street
Santa Barbara, CA 93101-4104
805-963-1426

ALA of Santa Clara–San Benito Counties
1469 Park Avenue
San Jose, CA 95126-2530
408-998-5864

ALA of Ventura County
2073 N. Oxnard Boulevard, Suite 400
Oxnard, CA 93030-2964
805-988-6023

COLORADO

ALA of Colorado
1600 Race Street
Denver, CO 80206-1198
303-388-4327

CONNECTICUT

ALA of Connecticut
45 Ash Street
East Hartford, CT 06108-3272
860-289-5401

DELAWARE

ALA of Delaware
1021 Gilpin Avenue, Suite 202
Wilmington, DE 19806-3280
302-655-7258

DISTRICT OF COLUMBIA

ALA of the District of Columbia
475 H Street NW
Washington, DC 20001-2617
202-682-5864

FLORIDA

ALA of Florida, Inc.
5526 Arlington Road
Jacksonville, FL 32211-5216
904-743-2933

ALA of Central Florida, Inc.
1333 W. Colonial Drive
Orlando, FL 32804-7133
407-425-5864

ALA of Gulfcoast Florida, Inc.
6170 Central Avenue
Saint Petersburg, FL 33707-1523
813-347-6133

ALA of South Florida, Inc.
2020 S. Andrews Avenue
Fort Lauderdale, FL 33316-3430
954-524-4657

ALA of Southeast Florida, Inc.
2701 N. Australian Avenue
West Palm Beach, FL 33407-4526
561-659-7644

GEORGIA

ALA of Georgia
2452 Spring Road
Smyrna, GA 30080-3862
770-434-5864

HAWAII

ALA of Hawaii
245 N. Kukui Street, Suite 100
Honolulu, HI 96817
808-537-5966

IDAHO/NEVADA

ALA of Idaho/Nevada
6119 Ridgeview Court, Suite 100
Reno, NV 89509
702-829-5864

ILLINOIS

ALA of Metropolitan Chicago
(Chicago and Cook Counties)
1440 W. Washington Boulevard
Chicago, IL 60607-1878
312-243-2000

ALA of Illinois
1 Christmas Seal Drive
Springfield, IL 62703
217-528-3441

ALA of Central Illinois
922 N. Sheridan Road
Peoria, IL 61606-1910
309-672-2290

ALA of DuPage & McHenry Counties
1749 S. Naperville Road, Suite 202
Wheaton, IL 60187
630-260-9600

ALA of North Central Illinois
402 Countryside Center
Yorkville, IL 60560
630-553-7000

INDIANA

ALA of Indiana
9410 Priority Way West Drive
Indianapolis, IN 46240-1470
317-573-3900

IOWA

ALA of Iowa
1025 Ashworth Road, Suite 410
West Des Moines, IA 50265-6600
515-224-0800

KANSAS

ALA of Kansas
4300 Drury Lane
Topeka, KS 66604-2419
913-272-9290

KENTUCKY

ALA of Kentucky
4100 Churchman Avenue
Louisville, KY 40215
502-363-2652

LOUISIANA

ALA of Louisiana, Inc.
2325 Severn Avenue, Suite 8
Metairie, LA 70001-6918
504-828-5864

MAINE

ALA of Maine
122 State Street
Augusta, ME 04330
207-622-6394

MARYLAND

ALA of Maryland
1840 York Road, Suites K–M
Timonium, MD 21093-5156
410-560-2120

MASSACHUSETTS

ALA of Massachusetts
1505 Commonwealth Avenue
Brighton, MA 02135-3605
617-787-5864

ALA of Greater Norfolk County
25 Spring Street
Walpole, MA 02081-4302
508-668-6729

ALA of Middlesex County
5 Mountain Road
P.O. Box 265
Burlington, MA 01803
617-272-2866

ALA of Western Massachusetts
393 Maple Street
Springfield, MA 01105
413-737-3506

MICHIGAN

ALA of Michigan
18860 W. Ten Mile Road
Southfield, MI 48075-2689
248-559-5100

MINNESOTA

ALA of Minnesota
490 Concordia Avenue
Saint Paul, MN 55103-2441
612-227-8014

ALA of Hennepin County
4220 Old Shakopee Road, #101
Bloomington, MN 55437-2951
612-885-0338

MISSISSIPPI

ALA of Mississippi
353 N. Mart Plaza
Jackson, MS 39206-5316
601-362-5453

MISSOURI

ALA of Eastern Missouri
1118 Hampton Avenue
Saint Louis, MO 63139-3196
314-645-5505

ALA of Western Missouri
2007 Broadway
Kansas City, MO 64108-2080
816-842-5242

MONTANA

(See ALA of the Northern Rockies)

NEBRASKA

ALA of Nebraska
7101 Newport Avenue, Suite 303
Omaha, NE 68152
402-572-3030

NEVADA

(See ALA of Idaho/Nevada)

NEW HAMPSHIRE

ALA of New Hampshire
456 Beech Street
Manchester, NH 03103
603-669-2411

NEW JERSEY

ALA of New Jersey
1600 Route 22 East
Union, NJ 07083-3407
908-687-9340

NEW MEXICO

ALA of New Mexico
216 Truman NE
Albuquerque, NM 87108
505-265-0732

NEW YORK STATE

ALA of New York State
8 Mountain View Avenue
Albany, NY 12205-2804
518-453-0172

ALA of Central New York
1620 Burnet Avenue
Syracuse, NY 13206
315-422-6142

ALA of Finger Lakes Region
1595 Elmwood Avenue
Rochester, NY 14620
716-442-4260

ALA of the Hudson Valley
35 Orchard Street
White Plains, NY 10603-3397
914-949-2150

ALA of Mid New York
311 Turner Street, Suite 415
Utica, NY 13501-1731
315-735-9225

ALA of Nassau-Suffolk
225 Wireless Boulevard
Hauppauge, NY 11788-3914
516-231-5864

ALA of Western New York
210 John Glenn Drive, #3
Buffalo, NY 14228
716-691-5864

NEW YORK CITY

ALA of Brooklyn
165 Cadman Plaza East, Room 300
Brooklyn, NY 11201-1484
718-624-8531

ALA of New York
(Manhattan/Bronx/Staten Island)
432 Park Avenue South, 8th Floor
New York, NY 10016
212-889-3370 Manhattan
718-966-6700 for Bronx
and Staten Island

ALA of Queens
112-25 Queens Boulevard
Forest Hills, NY 11375
718-263-5656

NORTH CAROLINA

ALA of North Carolina
1323 Capital Boulevard, Suite 102
Raleigh, NC 27603
919-832-8326
800-892-5650

NORTH DAKOTA

ALA of North Dakota
212 N. 2nd Street
Bismarck, ND 58501
701-223-5613

NORTHERN ROCKIES

ALA of the Northern Rockies
825 Helena Avenue
Helena, MT 59601
406-442-6556

OHIO

ALA of Ohio
1950 Arlingate Lane
Columbus, OH 43228-4102
614-279-1700

OKLAHOMA

ALA of Oklahoma
2805 E. Skelly Drive, Suite 806
Tulsa, OK 74105
918-747-3441

OREGON

ALA of Oregon
9320 SW Barbur Boulevard, Suite 140
Portland, OR 97219-5481
503-246-1997

PENNSYLVANIA

ALA of Pennsylvania
6041 Linglestown Road
Harrisburg, PA 17112-1208
717-541-5864

ALA of Central Pennsylvania
6041 Linglestown Road
Harrisburg, PA 17112-1208
717-541-5864

ALA of Lancaster & Berks Counties
630 Janet Avenue
Lancaster, PA 17601-4584
717-397-5203

ALA of the Lehigh Valley
2121 Cityline Road
Bethlehem, PA 18017-2100
610-867-4100

ALA of Northeast Pennsylvania
738 S. Maine Avenue
Scranton, PA 18504
717-346-1784 or 343-0987

ALA of Northwest Pennsylvania
352 W. 8th Street
Erie, PA 16502-1498
814-454-0109 or
800-352-0917 in local areas, outside
Erie County

ALA of Southeastern Pennsylvania
525 Plymouth Road, Suite 315
Plymouth Meeting, PA 19462
610-941-9595

ALA of South Central Pennsylvania
488 W. Market Street
York, PA 17404
717-845-5864

ALA of Western Pennsylvania
Cranberry Professional Park
201 Smith Drive
Cranberry Township, PA 16066
412-772-1750

PUERTO RICO

Asociación Puertorriqueña del Pulmón
P.O. Box 195247
San Juan, PR 00919-5247
787-765-5664

RHODE ISLAND

ALA of Rhode Island
10 Abbott Park Place
Providence, RI 02903-3700
401-421-6487

SOUTH CAROLINA

ALA of South Carolina
1817 Gadsden Street
Columbia, SC 29201-2392
803-779-5864

SOUTH DAKOTA

ALA of South Dakota
1212 W. Elkhorn Street, #1
Sioux Falls, SD 57104-0218
605-336-7222

TENNESSEE

ALA of Tennessee, Inc.
1808 West End Avenue, Suite 514
Nashville, TN 37203
615-329-1151

TEXAS

ALA of Texas
5926 Balcones Drive, Suite 100
Austin, TX 78731-4263
512-467-6753

UTAH

ALA of Utah
1930 S. 1100 East
Salt Lake City, UT 84106-2317
801-484-4456

VERMONT

ALA of Vermont
30 Farrell Street
South Burlington, VT 05403-6196
802-863-6817

VIRGINIA

ALA of Virginia
311 South Boulevard
Richmond, VA 23220-5705
804-355-3295

ALA of Northern Virginia
9735 Main Street
Fairfax, VA 22031-3798
703-591-4131

VIRGIN ISLANDS

ALA of the Virgin Islands
P.O. Box 974
Saint Thomas, VI 00804
809-774-8620

WASHINGTON

ALA of Washington
2625 Third Avenue
Seattle, WA 98121-1213
206-441-5100

WEST VIRGINIA

ALA of West Virginia
415 Dickinson Street
Charleston, WV 25301
304-342-6600

WISCONSIN

ALA of Wisconsin
150 S. Sunny Slope Road, Suite 105
Brookfield, WI 53005-6461
414-782-7833

WYOMING

(See ALA of the Northern Rockies)

Government Resources

National Asthma Education and Prevention Program
(Part of the National Heart, Lung, and Blood Institute)
P.O. Box 30105
Bethesda, MD 20824-0105
301-251-1222

National Institute of Allergy and Infectious Diseases
Building 31
Room 7A50
Bethesda, MD 20892
301-496-5717

Other Organizations

Asthma and Allergy Foundation of America
1125 15th St. NW
Suite 502
Washington, DC 20005
800-7-ASTHMA

Allergy and Asthma Network/Mothers of Asthmatics, Inc.
3554 Chain Bridge Road
Suite 200
Fairfax, VA 22030-2709
800-878-4403

American Academy of Allergy, Asthma & Immunology
61 E. Wells Street
Milwaukee, WI 53202
800-822-ASMA

American College of Allergy, Asthma and Immunology
800 E. Northwest Highway,
Suite 1080
Palatine, IL 60067
800-842-7777

Medic Alert Foundation
2323 Colorado
Turlock, CA 95382
800-432-5378

List of References

References in addition to American Lung Association publications and other materials.

BOOKS

Feldman, B. Robert, and David Carroll. *The Complete Book of Children's Allergies.* New York: Warner Books, 1986.

Hannaway, Paul J. *The Asthma Self-Help Book: How to Live a Normal Life in Spite of Your Condition.* Revised Second Edition. Rocklin, CA: Prima Publishing, 1992.

Klein, Gerald A., and Vicki Timerman. *Keys to Parenting the Asthmatic Child.* Hauppauge, NY: Baron's, 1994.

Plaut, Thomas F. *Children with Asthma: A Manual for Parents.* Second Edition. Amherst, MA: Pedipress, Inc., 1988.

Rapp, Doris. *Is This Your Child?* New York: Quill/William Morrow, 1991.

Sander, Nancy. *A Parent's Guide to Asthma: How You Can Help Your Child Control Asthma at Home, School, and Play.* New York: Plume, 1994.

Weinstein, Allan M. *Asthma: The Complete Guide to Self-Management of Asthma and Allergies for Patients and Their Families.* New York: Fawcett Crest, 1987.

Wood, Robert A. *Taming Asthma and Allergy by Controlling Your Environment: A Guide for Patients.* Baltimore: Asthma and Allergy Foundation of America, 1995.

Young, Stuart H., Bruce S. Dobozin, and Margret Miner. *Allergies: The Complete Guide to Diagnosis, Treatment, and Daily Management.* Yonkers, NY: Consumer Reports Books, 1991.

GOVERNMENT REPORTS

National Asthma Education and Prevention Program. *Report of the Second Expert Panel on the Guidelines for the Diagnosis and Management of Asthma,* 1997. Available online at the National Heart, Lung and Blood Institute website: http://www.nhlbi.nih.gov/nhlbi.htm.

National Asthma Education and Prevention Program. *Asthma in the Elderly: Considerations for Diagnosing and Managing Asthma in the Elderly.* Bethesda, MD: National Institutes of Health, NIH Publication No. 96-3662, 1996.

National Asthma Education Program. Expert Panel Report. *Executive Summary: Guidelines for the Diagnosis and Management of Asthma.* Bethesda, MD: National Institutes of Health, NIH Publication No. 94-3042A, 1994.

National Asthma Education Program. Report of the Working Group on Asthma and Pregnancy. *Executive Summary: Management of Asthma During Pregnancy.* Bethesda, MD: National Institutes of Health, NIH Publication No. 93-3279A, 1993.

Glossary

Airway twitchiness: The hallmark sign of asthma, indicating that the airways are prone to inflammation and constriction from exposure to an asthma promoter or trigger.

Allergen: Any substance that causes an allergy attack.

Allergic contact dermatitis: A rash that occurs when the skin is exposed to or comes into contact with certain allergens. The most common form of allergic contact dermatitis is from exposure to poison ivy.

Allergic rhinitis: Term for hay fever, the allergy to pollen, dust mites, and mold spores.

Alveoli: The inside end of the airway tree, consisting of air sacs within the lungs attached to the ends of tiny bronchioles, which hold and transfer oxygen to the bloodstream.

Anaphylaxis: A potentially fatal allergic reaction that affects the entire body.

Antihistamines: A class of drugs that block the reaction of histamine and are commonly used to treat allergies.

Asthma promoters: Conditions and substances, such as allergies, tobacco smoke, and colds and respiratory infections, that can lead to lasting inflammation in the airways and leave them prone to react faster or more severely to an asthma trigger.

Atopic (allergic) dermatitis: Also called atopic eczema, a skin rash that occurs after exposure to an allergen.

Atopic eczema: Also called atopic dermatitis, a skin rash that occurs after exposure to an allergen.

Beta-adrenergic drugs: Oral or inhaled drugs that quickly open constricted airways, easing wheezing and asthma attacks.

Beta agonist: Another name for beta-adrenergic drugs.

Bronchial tubes: The large main airways that carry air to the lungs.

Bronchioles: Small branches of the bronchial tubes within the lungs.

Bronchoconstriction: Narrowing of the bronchioles.

Bronchodilator: A drug that eases constriction in the airways.

Bronchoprovocation test: A test used to diagnose asthma in which drugs are used to mimic an asthma attack.

Bronchospasm: Tightening of the muscles surrounding the airways, making them narrow.

Burst treatment: A term used to define short, usually week-long treatments with oral steroids for severe asthma attacks.

Chronic inflammation: A term indicating that the lungs of people with asthma are always inflamed and thus prone to constriction and attacks of wheezing.

Chronic rhinitis: Persistent or chronic inflammation of the lining of the nose.

Corticosteroids: Inhaled, nasal, oral, or injectable drugs used to reduce inflammation in the lungs or nasal passages, thus reducing the severity and perhaps preventing many asthma and allergy attacks.

Cromolyn: An inhaled anti-inflammatory drug used principally by children and people with exercise-induced asthma to prevent attacks and lessen their severity. Nasal cromolyn often is used by people with hay fever to prevent allergy attacks.

Cytokines: A group of chemicals produced by cells in the body that can lead to airway inflammation and constriction.

Decongestants: A class of drugs used to relieve mucus, or congestion, in the nose or nasal passages.

Dry powder inhalers: Asthma inhalers that deliver an inhalation of dry powder medication rather than an aerosolized mist.

Environmental control: Steps to take to reduce levels of asthma triggers and promoters in the home, school, and work environments.

Exercise-induced asthma: A temporary narrowing of the airways, or bronchoconstriction, that occurs after strenuous exercise, and may affect people who do not have other forms of asthma.

Face masks: Devices on the ends of spacers or nebulizer tubes that attach to a child's face and ensure delivery of medication mist.

Food allergy: An allergic reaction to a food or food additive caused by the same IgE and mast cell reactions responsible for hay fever and other allergies.

Food intolerance: Stomach upset that is not related to a true allergy.

Food poisoning: A reaction to toxins, bacteria, or other parasites in contaminated foods.

Fungi: Mold plants that lack stems, many of whose spores are able to provoke asthma and allergy attacks.

Hay fever: An allergy to pollen, dust mites, and mold spores.

HEPA (High Efficiency Particulate Air) filter: An air filter that removes tiny particles and allergens from the air.

Histamine: One of the most important irritating chemicals released by mast cells; it is most responsible for the symptoms of allergy attacks.

Hives: An itchy swelling of the skin from an allergic reaction.

IgE: The antibody known as immunoglobulin gamma E, which is located on the surfaces of mast cells and is thought to latch on to allergens and stimulate mast cells to release chemicals that irritate the airways.

Immune system: The body system, made up of the bone marrow, thymus gland, and lymph nodes, that protects against disease and infections. An overactive immune system can lead to the development of allergic diseases, such as asthma, hay fever, and other allergies.

Immunotherapy: Injections or nasal sprays in which tiny amounts of allergens are given over time to reduce a person's sensitivity, or allergic reactions, to the substances.

Infectious rhinitis: Rhinitis caused by the common cold or flu.

Mediators: Chemicals released by mast cells that cause inflammatory reactions.

Metered-dose inhalers: Pocket-sized canisters and mouthpieces containing aerosolized asthma medications.

Mold: Any of various fungi having spores, many of which are capable of causing asthma and allergy attacks.

Mucus: A protective, cleansing fluid produced by glands that can clog the airway tree when overproduced.

Nebulizers: A small air compressor used to deliver aerosolized asthma medications to children too young to master the use of metered-dose inhalers.

Nedocromil: An inhaled anti-inflammatory drug typically used as an alternative to inhaled corticosteroids to prevent attacks and lessen their severity.

Peak flow meter: A hand-held device for use at home to measure peak flow rate.

Peak flow rate: A measurement of the openness of the airways.

Pharmacologic food reaction: A reaction to a food additive or naturally occurring chemical in food, such as the jitters from the caffeine in coffee.

RAST: A blood test used to determine levels of IgE antibodies, high levels of which may indicate the existence of allergies or asthma.

Retraction: A phenomenon in which a person with asthma struggles so hard for air that the chest may appear concave and the ribs may show.

Rhinitis: Inflammation of the lining of the nose, leading to sneezing and a runny or itchy nose.

Sensitization: The process by which people with a predisposition to develop allergies become sensitive to specific allergens through repeated exposure to the substances.

Skin test: Tests in which tiny amounts of allergens are scratched into the surface of the skin to determine which can cause an allergic reaction.

Spacers: Tubelike devices attached to the end of the mouthpieces of metered-dose inhalers to collect the medication mist, thus more accurately dispersing the mist in the lungs and aiding young children in the use of inhalers.

Theophylline: An oral or inhaled bronchodilator, used less frequently since the advent of beta-adrenergic drugs.

Trachea: The tube connecting the mouth to the bronchial tubes.

Tryptase: A chemical produced by the body that is elevated following an allergy attack.

Wheal: The small round skin rash that develops after a positive allergy skin test.

Wheeze: A high-pitched whistling noise made upon breathing and caused when air moves through constricted airways.

Index